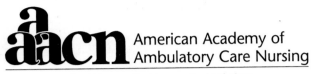

American Academy of Ambulatory Care Nursing

Real Nurses. Real Issues. Real Solutions.

Ambulatory Care Nursing Orientation and Competency Assessment Guide

2010 - 2nd Edition

Linda Brixey, RN
Editor

Copyright © 2010
American Academy of Ambulatory Care Nursing
East Holly Avenue, Box 56
Pitman, NJ 08071-0056

1-800-AMB-NURS
Web site: www.aaacn.org

0-9819379-2-2

D1075687

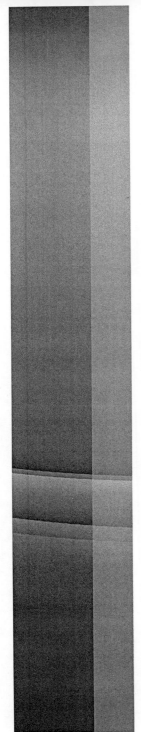

Ambulatory Care Nursing Orientation and Competency Assessment Guide

2010 - 2nd Edition

Linda Brixey, RN
Editor

Managing Editor: Katie R. Brownlow, ELS
Layout & Design Specialist: Darin Peters
Art Director: Jack M. Bryant

Publication Management:
Anthony J. Jannetti, Inc.
East Holly Avenue, Box 56
Pitman, NJ 08071-0056
Phone: 856-256-2300
Fax: 856-589-7463
Web site: www.ajj.com

Disclaimer
The authors, contributors, editors, and publishers of this book have made serious efforts to ensure that treatments, practices, and procedures are accurate and conform to standards accepted at the time of publication. Due to constant changes in information resulting from continuing research and clinical experience, reasonable differences in opinions among authorities, unique aspects of individual clinical situations, and the possibility of human error in preparing such a publication, the reader should exercise individual judgment when making a clinical decision, and if necessary, consult and compare information from other authorities, professionals, or sources.

Suggested citation:
Brixey, L. (Ed.). (2010). *Ambulatory care nursing orientation and competency assessment guide* (2nd ed.). Pitman, NJ: American Academy of Ambulatory Care Nursing.

Table of Contents

    A-1.   Delegation of Tasks and Procedures
    A-2.   Environmental Management
    A-2(1). Environmental Safety
    A-3.   Ethics
    A-4.   Informatics and HIPAA
    A-5.   Informatics Application
    A-6.   Audit Tool for Blood Pressure
    A-7.   Audit Tool for Documentation

Table of Contents

Preface

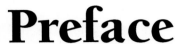

The health care climate and the economic environment provide challenges for ambulatory care nurses and validate the need for up-to-date resources to maintain quality care and meet organizational needs. The AAACN Staff Education Special Interest Group, with the help of other member experts, revised and updated the *Ambulatory Care Nursing Orientation and Competency Guide*.

The objectives in revising the guide were to:
- Assure the updated resource materials clearly describe the attributes of the ambulatory care environment, nursing requirements for quality patient care, and specific role dimensions of competent nurses.
- Promote standardized competencies for ambulatory care nurses.
- Further augment existing organizational systems, tools, and processes that distinguish ambulatory care nursing as a specialty and professional entity.

This guide presents fundamental competencies to direct the orientation process for new staff. The information can also be used to evaluate existing staff. The competencies are designed for registered nurses and other staff as regulated by their practice acts and job descriptions. The authors encourage readers to integrate the concept of competency in designing an orientation plan. This publication will be a valuable guide in this endeavor.

Orientation plans should reflect the individual needs of the organization and the employee. The guide identifies multiple skills from which an organization can choose to design a competency-based orientation.

Chapter 1: "Putting It All Together" more completely describes how to use this guide.

Chapters 2-5 describe competencies and their elements that may be used when designing an orientation plan. These chapters have been broken into four domains of nursing practice: Organizational/Systems, Clinical Nursing, Professional Nurse Role, and Telehealth Nursing Practice.

The authors expanded the content of the guide to meet the needs of nurse educators and nurses new to ambulatory care. This edition of the guide includes competency and role descriptions for the ambulatory care nurse educator. A toolkit to facilitate transition into ambulatory care directs the user in what tools are available and how to best use them when transitioning into ambulatory care.

The appendices provide examples of how various organizations have identified and incorporated competencies into their plan. Appendix A provides examples of organizational competency assessment tools; Appendix B provides nursing practice competencies, and Appendix C provides tools for professional practice. Appendix D provides orientation plan examples, and Appendix E provides examples of orientation competency validation checklists.

Contributors

Carol Ann Attwood, MLS, AHIP, MPH, RN, C
Mayo Clinic
Scottsdale, AZ

Carol Brautigam, MSN, RN
Kaiser Permanente
Denver, CO

Linda Brixey, RN
Kelsey Seybold Clinic
Houston, TX

Lenora J. Flint, MSN, MS, RN, PHN, CNS
Kaiser Permanente
Baldwin Park, CA

DiAnn Hughes, BA, ABRM
Kaiser Permanente
Baldwin Park, CA

Jane Hummer, BSN, MPH, RN-BC, COHN-S
University of Iowa Hospital and Clinics
Iowa City, IA

Anne Jessie, MSN, BSN, RN
Carilion Clinic
Roanoke, VA

Kathy Kesner, MS, RN, CNS
University of Colorado Hospital
Aurora, CO

Caroline Koehler, MSN, RN
Kaiser Permanente
Denver, CO

Maj Carla Leeseberg, MSN/Ed, RN-BC
U.S. Air Force
San Antonio, TX

Catherine Liebau, MSN, RN
Community Memorial Medical Commons
Menomonee Falls, WI

Wanda Mayo, BSN, RN, CPN
Children's Medical Center Dallas
Arlington, TX

CDR Terrie C. McSween, NC, USN
United States Navy
Groton, CT

Leslie Morris, BSN, RN
Kelsey Seybold Clinic
Houston, TX

Sue Olsson, BSN, RN-BC
University of Michigan
Ann Arbor, MI

Donna Pforr, BSN, EdM
Carl Clinic
Fischer, IL

Marianne Sherman, RN, MS,C
University of Colorado Hospital
Aurora, CO

Charlene Williams, BSN, RN, BC, MBA
Duke University Health System
Durham, NC

Reviewers

Col. Carol Andrews, MS, BSN, RN, RN-C,
BC, CNA
U.S. Air Force
San Antonio, TX

Irene Berg, MSN, RN-BC
Mayo Clinic
Rochester, MN

Wanda Mayo, BSN, RN, CPN
Children's Medical Center Dallas
Arlington, TX

Kathryn Scheidt, MSN, RN, CPHQ
McKesson Health Solutions
Broomfield, CO

Lynn Smith-Cronin, BSN, RN
Kelsey Seybold Clinic
Houston, TX

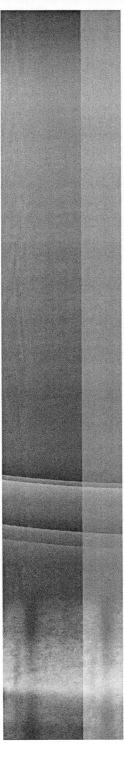

Acknowledgments

The American Academy of Ambulatory Care Nursing (AAACN) would like to acknowledge the inspiration and creative forces for the *Ambulatory Care Nursing Orientation and Competency Assessment Guide*.

Thanks to Betty Cody, Marianne Sherman, and Lenora Flint, who chaired the Staff Education Special Interest Group (Staff Ed SIG) during the development of the original book.

During this revision, Carol Brautigam, Carla Leeseberg, and Donna Pforr played an important role as SIG chairs in guiding the Staff Ed SIG through the process. Catherine Liebau volunteered to chair the Guide's revision.

This edition of the Guide includes two new sections: *Nurse Educator Competencies* and *Resources for the Nurse Transitioning to Ambulatory Care.*

Lenora Flint and DiAnn Hughes developed the general outline for the *Educator Competencies*. Members of the Staff Ed SIG used the outline to develop the new section on staff educator competencies. Lenora and DiAnn also created a template to update the original Guide, which the Staff Ed SIG reviewed and accepted as value added to the tool.

Resources for the Nurse Transitioning to Ambulatory Care was the "brain child" of Pamela Delmonte. Catherine Liebau used Pamela's research to create this section.

Thank you to all the contributors and reviewers who volunteered their time and expertise to the creation of this excellent resource for ambulatory care nurses.

Linda Brixey, RN
Editor and AAACN Board Liaison to
Staff Education Special Interest Group (SIG)
*Ambulatory Care Nursing Orientation and
Competency Assessment Guide (2nd ed.)*

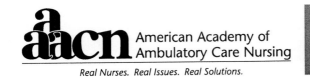

IDENTITY STATEMENT:

The American Academy of Ambulatory Care Nursing (AAACN) is the association of professional nurses and associates who identify ambulatory care practice as essential to the continuum of accessible, high-quality, and cost-effective health care.

MISSION AND CORE PURPOSE:

Advance the art and science of ambulatory care nursing.

CORE VALUES:

The following values guide member and the organization vision, actions, and relationships:
1) Responsible health care delivery for individuals and communities;
2) Visionary and accountable leadership;
3) Productive partnerships and alliances;
4) Diversity;
5) Continual advancement of professional ambulatory care nursing practice;
6) Collaborative professional community.

GOALS:

➤ **KNOWLEDGE** – AAACN will be the recognized source for knowledge in ambulatory care nursing.

➤ **EDUCATION** – Nurses will have the leadership skills and capabilities to articulate, promote, and practice nursing successfully in an ambulatory care setting.

➤ **ADVOCACY** – The healthcare community will recognize and value ambulatory care nursing.

➤ **COMMUNITY** – Ambulatory care nurses will have a supportive and collaborative community in which to share professional interests, experience, and practice.

ABOUT AAACN:

AAACN (formerly the American Academy of Ambulatory Nursing Administration) was founded in 1978 as a not for profit, educational forum. In 1993, the organization's name was changed to the American Academy of Ambulatory Care Nursing (AAACN). Membership was broadened to include nurses in direct practice, education, and research roles as well as those in management and administration. Today, membership is open to nurses and other professionals interested in ambulatory care nursing. Corporations and individual corporate representatives are also welcomed as members.

Ambulatory practice settings include universities, medical centers, HMOs, group practices, urgent care centers, physician office settings, hospital-based ambulatory care settings, military, community health, and others. The Academy serves as a voice for ambulatory care nurses across the continuum of health care delivery and has membership in the Nursing Organizations Alliance (NOA). The Alliance provides a forum for nursing organizations to dialogue, collaborate, and facilitate policy formulation on professional practice and national health.

MEMBERSHIP BENEFITS:

Academy membership benefits include discounted rates to the AAACN National Preconference and Conference offering multiple practice innovations, industry exhibits, and numerous networking opportunities. Other benefits include distance learning programs, special member rates on publications and the fee to take the ANCC ambulatory care nursing certification exam; the bimonthly newsletter – *Viewpoint*; subscription to **one** of four journals – *Nursing Economic$*, *MEDSURG Nursing*, *Dermatology Nursing*, or *Pediatric Nursing*; opportunity to join a special interest group in the area of: Leadership, Patient Education, Pediatrics, Staff Education, Telehealth Nursing Practice, Veterans Affairs, and Tri-Service Military; awards and scholarship programs; access to national experts and colleagues through AAACN's online membership directory, monthly E-newsletter, E-mail discussion lists, an Expert Panel, Web site **aaacn.org**; and online Career Center.

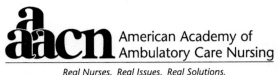

AAACN PUBLICATIONS/EDUCATION RESOURCES:

➤ *Ambulatory Care Nurse Staffing: An Annotated Bibliography*
➤ *Ambulatory Care Nursing Certification Review Course Syllabus*
➤ *Ambulatory Care Nursing Certification Review Course CD-ROM*
➤ *Ambulatory Care Nursing Orientation and Competency Assessment Guide*, 2nd Edition
➤ *Ambulatory Care Nursing Review Questions*
➤ *Core Curriculum for Ambulatory Care Nursing*, 2nd Edition
➤ *Scope and Standards of Practice for Professional Ambulatory Care Nursing*, 8th Edition
➤ *Telehealth Nursing Practice Administration and Practice Standards*, 4th Edition
➤ *Telehealth Nursing Practice Core Course (TNPCC) CD-ROM*
➤ *Telehealth Nursing Practice Essentials*
➤ *Telehealth Nursing Practice Resource Directory*

AAACN COURSES:

• Ambulatory Care Nursing Certification Review Course*
• Telehealth Nursing Practice Core Course (TNPCC)*
    *Both courses can be presented at your location.

ANNUAL CONFERENCE:

AAACN provides cutting-edge information and education at its annual conference, usually held in the month of March or April. Nurses from across the country as well as international colleagues come together to network, learn from each other, and share knowledge and skills. Renowned speakers in the field of ambulatory care present topics of current interest offering over 28 contact hours. An Exhibit Hall featuring the products and services of vendors serving the ambulatory care and telehealth community provides information and resources to attendees.

LIVE AUDIO SEMINARS:

Monthly continuing education on timely topics is convenient for nurses and cost-effective.

CERTIFICATION:

AAACN values the importance of certification and promotes achieving this level of competency through its educational products to prepare nurses to take the ambulatory care nursing certification examination. AAACN strongly encourages all telehealth nurses to become certified in ambulatory care nursing. Because telehealth nurses provide nursing care to patients who are in an ambulatory setting, they must possess the knowledge and competencies to appropriately provide ambulatory care. Ambulatory certification is and will continue to be the gold standard credential for any nursing position within ambulatory care.

CORPORATE COLLABORATIONS:

Together, working with corporate colleagues, AAACN continues to advance the delivery of ambulatory care to patients. AAACN is open to alliances or collaborations with corporate industry to achieve mutual goals. Corporations are encouraged to contact the national office to suggest ways AAACN can work with them to advance the practice of ambulatory care nursing.

American Academy of Ambulatory Care Nursing

East Holly Avenue, Box 56
Pitman, NJ 08071-0056
Phone: 800-262-6877/Fax: 856-589-7463
Email: aaacn@ajj.com
Web site: www.aaacn.org

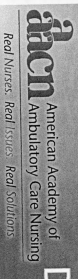

aaacn

American Academy of
Ambulatory Care Nursing

Real Nurses. Real Issues. Real Solutions.

Do you practice in a setting

other than

a traditional
inpatient setting?

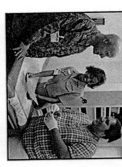
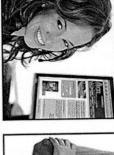
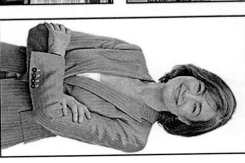

...then you are an

ambulatory care nurse!

If you work in a:

- Medical office
- Telehealth/call center
- School
- Government institution
- Military clinic
- Managed care/HMO/PPO
- Group practice or health center
- Home health setting
- University, community, or private hospital

⬤ Good news

The American Academy of Ambulatory Care Nursing (AAACN) has been helping nurses like you achieve extraordinary career success because our programs and benefits are designed *specifically for your needs.*

Become part of a nurturing community that helps you fast-track your professional success.

Join AAACN today!

To find out more, visit
www.aaacn.org
or call 800-AMB-NURS

Introduction

Linda Brixey, RN
Marianne Sherman RN, MS,C

In the ambulatory care setting, individuals involved in providing nursing care want to ensure the safe and competent practice of nursing. Therefore, healthcare organizations, regulatory agencies, professional organizations, and nurse educators often develop standards and approaches to the acquisition and maintenance of competencies. The term *competency*, although widely used, may have different applications in various organizations.

For instance, The Joint Commission states that "competency assessment can be accomplished through a variety of methods including the assessment of information from current and previous employers, collecting peer feedback, verifying certification and licensure, reviewing test results with a written or oral competency, and observation of skills. The assessment must be thorough and focus on the particular competency needs for the clinical staff's assignment. Use of a self-assessment, such as a skills checklist, as the sole assessment method does not constitute a competency assessment" (JCAHO, 2004). According to their statement, an ongoing assessment program should be conducted to maintain competent staff members that provide quality patient care. The program also assists in matching applicants to open positions and ensures ongoing assessment of staff competency from initial review through annual reviews.

Donna Wright, a staff development specialist and nationally recognized expert in the development of competency assessment programs, defines competency as "the application of knowledge, skills and behaviors that are needed to fulfill organization, departmental and work setting requirements in the varied circumstances of the real world" (Wright, 1998). Similarly, The American Academy of Ambulatory Care Nursing (AAACN), in its *Core Curriculum for Ambulatory Care Nursing*, defines *competence* as "having the ability to demonstrate the technical, critical thinking, and interpersonal skills necessary to perform one's job" (Laughlin, 2006, p. 419).

These definitions reflect that competency is an ongoing process based upon organizational standards. Assessing staff competency begins at the time of interviewing and hiring, continuing through orientation and as an ongoing assessment of performance. Competency programs in ambulatory care settings should include a definition of the competency to be assessed, criteria and assessment methods, frequency of assessment, and actions to be taken if the individual does not meet competency expectations. Joyce Johnson's competency model (see Figure 1) provides a chart illustrating the progression of competency from hire through professional development.

The *Scope and Standards of Practice for Professional Ambulatory Care Nursing* direct ambulatory care nurses to "collaborate with appropriate department and other professionals in developing integrated systems that support ambulatory care delivery" (AAACN, 2010, p. 19). Collaboration with nursing staff and relevant professional resources can assist in the development of clearly written standards and criteria for competency for all clinical staff and assistive personnel working under the supervision of ambulatory care nurses.

Competency is a team effort comprised of individual nurses, employers, educators, professional organizations, and regulatory bodies.

A variety of methods may be utilized to measure competency. In the section on *Staff Educator Competencies*, descriptions of methods and tools are listed that measure one or more domains of competency: post-tests, return demonstration, case studies, observation of daily work, peer reviews, mock surveys, QI monitors, presentations, discussion groups, exemplars, and self-assessment. By measuring baseline competency through the use of various domains, the progression of skills acquisition can be measured.

- *Novice:* Can undertake the skill, but must be supervised/checked by a validator. Can complete the skill elements but needs more than the usual amount of time to do so and requires assistance from appropriate persons. May need to review the policy/procedure, but needs minimal prompting.
- *Independent:* Undertakes the skill easily, readily, within time frames, without any assistance or prompting.
- *Expert:* Can teach the skill and is a resource to others. Has in-depth understanding of the skill and problem-solving. Works at maximum level of efficiency and confidence. Functions as a trainer or validator in the department for the skill.
- *Not met:* Cannot undertake the skill. Does not or is unable to perform the skill despite following policy/procedure or given assistance/ prompting. Continues to make the same mistakes.

Competency validation begins during orientation in the classroom with skills labs and moves to the clinical setting using actual patients. The AAACN nursing conceptual framework provides a model for competency validation (AAACN, 2010) (see Figure 2). It recognizes the broad scope of ambulatory practice settings providing patient care. This is identified as the Internal Environment. The *Internal Environment* is the primary focus of an orientation. We also need to take into consideration the *External Environment*. These external factors can include, but are not

Figure 1.
Johnson's Competency Model

Raising the Bar of Performance

Assumptions:
Careful hiring practices will result in employees who are a good "fit" with the job and organization.
Orientation and continuing education are key retention strategies.
Validating competency improves competence and provides a mechanism for corrective action.
Providing feedback and targeted education/training helps the employee improve performance.
Creating a professional portfolio (requiring staff reflection on experiences) improves performance.

Anticipated Outcomes:
All employees will perform the responsibilities of their position in a skillful and excellent manner.
All employees will make sound judgements.
All employees will provide and model excellence in customer service; they will go the extra mile.
Collectively, this will result in raising the bar of performance and improving organizational
effectiveness and outcomes.
As a result, we will become the healthcare of choice and the employer of choice.

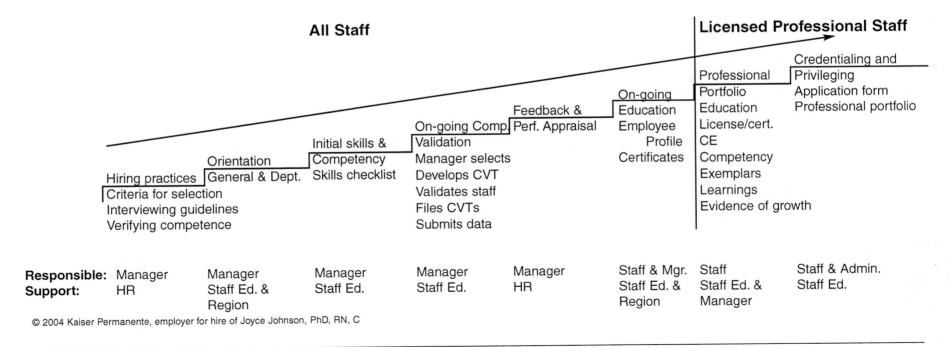

© 2004 Kaiser Permanente, employer for hire of Joyce Johnson, PhD, RN, C

limited to, the surrounding community population with its needs, perceptions, and resources; federal, state, and local laws and regulations; regulatory agencies; financial reimbursement systems; and technology (i.e., diagnostic and treatment technologies as well as the information systems that support and coordinate patient care through virtual information exchange).

This book is comprised of three sections: Staff orientation and competency program content, competencies of the staff educator, and tools for transitioning to ambulatory care.

Section 1

The first section relates to the specifics for building a comprehensive orientation and competency program for an organization or department. It describes the knowledge and skills associated with the dimensions of performance. Organizations need to assess what nursing skills should be incorporated into an orientation plan to prepare the nurse to provide competent and safe patient care in positions the nurse is to fill. The authors have added a *Definition, Key Action Tips,* and an *Example* for each dimension to facilitate implementation by the user.

Section 2

The second section is oriented to the Staff Educator's competencies. This section defines what competencies are needed by the Educator. Chapter 6 includes skills related to the leadership and consultant roles. The next chapters outline the tools and processes used to plan, build, and validate educational programs. This section provides a description of how to develop an atmosphere that facilitates the student's success through an appropriate learning environment and ongoing program evaluations. The Staff Educator also needs to continually expand his or her professional knowledge through self-development.

Section 3

The third section provides a tool box of tips and resources to transition a nurse new to the ambulatory care setting. This section helps identify clinical and administrative resources needed for successful ambulatory care nursing practice.

Many times, tools and information can be tailored to fit a staffing mix led by RNs, and including LPN/LVN and medical assistants. Nursing leaders enforce identified scope of practices for each level of caregiver as defined by the state and in alignment with the goals of the organization when developing the orientation template.

Ambulatory care services and facilities continue to evolve, necessitating increased numbers of nurses. Recruitment and retention of competent and dedicated ambulatory care staff is fiercely competitive, time-consuming and expensive. In today's market, nurses are offered and closely scrutinize lucrative work packages, however the HR data from exit interviews tells us these same nurses are equally, if not more, responsive to facilities offering comprehensive orientation programs.

AAACN envisions a planned orientation for ambulatory nurses to improve the nurse's understanding of ambulatory care. The orientation provided by managers, educators, and preceptors with demonstrated ambulatory competencies assure the value and future of the ambulatory nurse.

References

American Academy of Ambulatory Care Nursing (AAACN). (2010). *Scope and standards of practice for professional ambulatory care nursing* (8th ed.) Pitman, NJ: Author.

Joint Commission on Accreditation of Healthcare Organizations, The (JCAHO). (2004). *Assessing and improving staff competence* (CD-ROM). Oakbrook Terrace, IL: The Joint Commission Resources.

Laughlin, C.B. (Ed.). (2006). *Core curriculum for ambulatory care nursing* (2nd ed.). Pitman, NJ: American Academy of Ambulatory Care Nursing.

Wright, D. (1998). *The ultimate guide to competency assessment in healthcare* (2nd ed.). Eau Claire, WI: Professional Education Systems, Inc.

Additional Reading

Enstrum, S. (2001). The state board of nursing and its role in continued competency. *The Journal of Continuing Education in Nursing, 32*(3), 118-125.

Figure 2.
Ambulatory Care Nursing Conceptual Framework Diagram

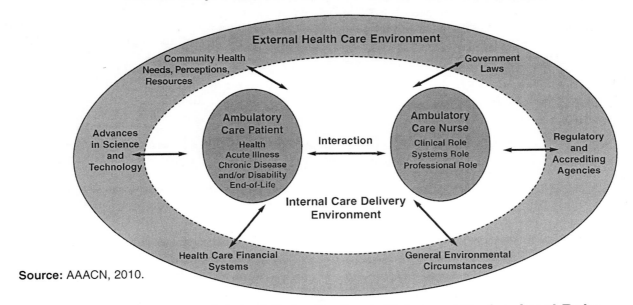

Source: AAACN, 2010.

Descriptors for Clinical Role, Systems Role, and Professional Role:

Clinical Nursing Role	Organizational/Systems Role	Professional Role
Assess patient problems and concerns	Administer and coordinate resources	Practice according to professional, ethical, and organizational standards
Critically analyze and integrate subjective and objective data	Direct clinical and organizational activities and workflows	Evidence-based practice
Identify problems and pertinent goals	Practice/office issues: staffing, staff development, workload and competency concerns	Evaluate outcomes
Plan appropriate nursing care	Workplace regulatory compliance (EEOC, OSHA)	Life-long expansion of ambulatory nursing knowledge and skills
Implement evidence-based nursing intervention	Risk management	Clinical quality improvement
Evaluate patient outcomes	Healthcare fiscal management (reimbursement and coding)	Leadership skills within healthcare
Advocacy: compassion, caring, and emotional support that is culturally competent and relevant	Legal and regulatory issues	Provider self-care
Refer patient to optimal health services	Organizational cultural competency	Priority management/delegation/supervision
Patient education: health promotion, preventing disease and complications	Health informatics	
Telehealth practice services	Conflict management	
Clinical procedures: perform appropriate nursing measures	Structuring customer-focused systems	
Consulting and collaboration with colleagues	Advocacy (inter-organizational and community)	
Careful and complete documentation of care	Ongoing political/entrepreneurial skills	
Protocol development/usage		

Putting It All Together: The Orientation Plan

Marianne Sherman, RN, MS,C

Finding skilled ambulatory nurses is a challenge. Some attribute this to the nursing shortage, while some argue that nursing schools inadequately teach the concepts of ambulatory nursing. Although nurses may use the same basic skills in various settings (such as collaboration, critical thinking, and assessment), how these skills are carried out in the ambulatory setting is unique (see Table 1). For example, documentation of care in ambulatory care nursing builds on each encounter and is longitudinal, while acute care is built on that admission. The ambulatory nurse is expected to make rapid assessments over the phone and in person for as many as 50 patients in a day. In light of these differences, an orientation for a nurse to a new nursing position in ambulatory care is not only worthwhile but necessary, regardless of how "seasoned" that nurse is.

The goal of an orientation plan for a nurse is to ensure the new employee has the skills and knowledge to deliver safe, ethical, and competent patient care. Orientation plays a key role in reducing employee turnover, contributing to patient safety, and ensuring a competently trained staff. The Joint Commission (2004) found that 63% of sentinel events are the result of little or no orientation to a new job or position. In addition, poor training and orientation is linked to a 15% turnover rate the first year at a great cost to the employer (Marcum & West, 2004). The chapters in this book were developed to assist educators, managers, organizations, and others in developing an effective competency-based orientation plan for their nursing staff.

Planning the Orientation

The *Core Curriculum for Ambulatory Care Nursing* (Laughlin, 2006) defines orientation as a planned process for introducing a new employee to the work setting and assessing the ability of the individual to perform basic job requirements.

Literature supports an orientation plan that is competency-based and flexible enough to meet the individual learning needs of the employee while supporting the mission and vision of the organization. A plan for a nurse transferring from another ambulatory setting and a nurse transitioning to ambulatory care for the first time will look different, but all plans are grounded in the standards of practice.

Components of an orientation plan can be identified and designed using various frameworks such as the nursing process (Alspach, 1996). Orientation plans should include an assessment to identify needs and assist with planning, implementation, and evaluation (Dignan & Carr, 1992). Orientation plans move from a global overview of the organization into job-specific competencies (see example in Table 2). An overview of the organization is a good starting point, but is inadequate in meeting the needs of the new employee in understanding the job duties and assessing the competencies required of the new position. The orientation plan may include ongoing training needs identified during this orientation phase. Orientation plans build on the competencies of the new employee and should always include an evaluation component. Examples of tools and processes which can be used to plan the orientation education and validate

Table 1.
Difference Between Nursing Role in Ambulatory and Inpatient Settings

Aspect of Role	Inpatient Practice	Ambulatory Practice
Treatment episode	Inpatient admission	Visit or phone encounter
Observation mode	Direct and continuous	Episodic, often using patient as informant
Management and treatment plan	By nurse with input from patient and family	By patient or family with input from the nurse
Primary intervention mode	Direct	Consultative
Organizational presence of nursing	Nurse-managed department	May or may not be formal structure for nursing
Workload variability and intensity	Determined by bed capacity and admission criteria	Theoretically determined by scheduling system

Source: Reprinted from Hastings, 2006.

Table 2.
Example of an Orientation Plan for the Clinical Nurse

Organizational ⟶ Divisional ⟶ Department/clinic specifics ⟶ Job specifics

Organizational	Division	Department	Job-Specific Skills		
Assessment and evaluation of employee	Ongoing assessment	Completes the assessment/evaluation process and initiates an orientation plan (see Appendix D)	Ongoing assessment and evaluation All new nurses will read the article "Transitioning from Acute Care to Ambulatory Care" (Swan, 2007)		
Human Resources/Professional Expectations	Job description	Essential job duties	Organizational role	Nursing practice Read article on transitioning to ambulatory care (Swan, 2007)	Professional practice
Mandatory (such as fire, safety, JCAHO, HIPAA, CPR)	Professional role expectations Safety/environment of care	Policies and procedures related to safety, environmental control, and infection control	Environment competency (see Appendix A-2)	Leapfrog Safety Initiatives (visit www.aaacn.org, click on "Links," then "Leapfrog")	*Core Curriculum for Ambulatory Care Nursing* (Laughlin, 2006) Read chapters 1-7
Mission, Vision, Values	Division goals and mission	Department scope of practice	*Core Curriculum for Ambulatory Care Nursing* (Laughlin, 2006) Read chapters 12-16	AAACN *ViewPoint* article "Achieving Evidence-Based Practice in Ambulatory Care Nursing" (Greenberg & Pyle, 2004)	*Scope and Standards of Practice for Professional Ambulatory Care Nursing* (AAACN, 2010) Read and review all chapters
Compliance Organizational charts	Organization of division	Organization and list of staff	*Core Curriculum for Ambulatory Care Nursing* (Laughlin, 2006) Read chapters 8-11	Clinical Nurse Study (see Appendix B-5)	*Ambulatory Care Nursing Certification Review Course* (CD-ROM) (AAACN, 2009)
Organizational charts Organizational skills CPR	Specific skill training (computers, emergency equipment)	Department-specific skills and equipment: point of care testing	*Telehealth Nursing Practice Essentials* (Espensen, 2009) Read chapters 1-6	Telehealth Nursing Practice (see Appendix B-4)	*Telehealth Nursing Administration and Practice Standards* (AAACN, 2007) Read and review

competencies are located in the appendix section of the book.

The book includes a section on the *Nurse Educator*. Chapter 7 describes how to plan education and validate programs. A nurse's culture, generation, and past experience will influence the plan and teaching modalities. Chapter 8 stresses the importance of the learning environment. Guidance is provided to identify the best teaching modalities, matching the needs of your organization and those of the learner.

The section of the book on *Transitioning to Ambulatory Care* presents a model for orienting a nurse who is new to the ambulatory care work setting. The section can be used as a guide for the nurse to seek appropriate resources for a successful transition to the ambulatory care setting.

Assessment

During the orientation process, the new employee's skills and competencies are assessed and an individual plan designed to meet the needs of the nurse in relation to the requirements of the position. Orientation assessment tools usually include a self-assessment component. Selection of training, education, and competency validation tools need to support the identified needs of the orientee and the organization. Examples of these tools are located in the appendices of this book.

Using the chapters on the *Ambulatory Nursing Roles*, specific job competencies can be selected which meet the requirements of the position. Examples of a needs assessment can be found in the section of the section of the book entitled *Nurse Educator Competencies*. These chapters discuss topics to consider during this assessment process such as evidence-based practice, community standards, program participants, etc.

Implementation

Once the topics for orientation are identified, the method for training is planned. For example, sedation training may be done by a self-paced computer training program with validation of specific skills accomplished in the clinical department. Methods used for training are instructor-led classes either on site or remote, self-paced modules of instruction, checklists, games, and computer-based programs. McConnell (1998) stated that "multisensory stimulation is best for increasing skill acquisition and retaining information." Documentation of orientation should include the topic, competency, and method used for validation (see examples in Appendices B-3 and E-1). The use of a preceptor assigned to orient a new employee has been discussed frequently in the literature as an effective method to socialize, educate, and role model the professional practice during the orientation process.

Most orientation plans include:
- A welcome
- Description of the culture (mission and vision)
- Description of who they are (organizational chart)
- Professional expectations
- Human Resources components
- Policy and procedures
- Skill assessment and training
- Pertinent information about safety, infection control, cultural diversity, ethics, and patient rights

Evaluation

Staff educators recognize the importance of ongoing evaluation and feedback related to the employee's ability to perform his or her skills. This can be achieved by weekly evaluations, peer review, audits, tests, performance evaluations, and other evaluation methods. Documentation of the orientation progress needs to be part of the employee's orientation plan and official record. Validation of an employee's ability to perform the competencies required of the job needs to occur before the employee delivers care independently.

Now You Begin...

Begin your plan by deciding what components, skills, and knowledge the nurse needs in order to perform his or her new job. Using the chapters on the ambulatory nursing roles, identify the needed skills. Plan how to orient and train the component and skills by using the educator competencies as a guide and designing a template for the plan. Select the methods to be used for validation. Assign a preceptor to train and socialize the employee. The examples in the Appendix illustrate various tools that are used for these processes. In addition, a list of resources is available on the AAACN Web site (www.aaacn.org).

Document the training, periodically evaluate the employee's progress, and provide feedback to the new employee. At the end of the orientation, the documented paperwork should include:
- Organizational and division orientation
- Department orientation that includes orientation to the safety within the department
- Signed job description
- Competency assessment and documentation
- Evaluation of progress

Utilizing a consistent approach in orienting new nursing staff will assist you in developing a competency-based orientation plan that is grounded in the standards of practice.

References

Alspach, J.G. (1996). *Designing competency assessment programs: A handbook for nursing and health-related profession.* Pensacola, FL: National Nursing Staff Development Organization.

American Academy of Ambulatory Care Nursing (AAACN). (2007). *Telehealth nursing administration and practice standards.* Pitman, NJ: Author.

American Academy of Ambulatory Care Nursing (AAACN). (2009). *Certification review course* (CD-ROM). Pitman, NJ: Author.

American Academy of Ambulatory Care Nursing (AAACN). (2010). *Scope and standards of practice for professional ambulatory care nursing* (8th ed.) Pitman, NJ: Author.

Dignan, M.B., & Carr, P.A. (1992). *Program planning for health education and promotion* (2nd ed.). Philadelphia: Lea and Febiger.

Espensen, M. (Ed.) (2009). *Telehealth nursing practice essentials.* Pitman, NJ: American Academy of Ambulatory Care Nursing.

Greenberg, M., & Pyle, B. (2004). Achieving evidence-based practice in ambulatory care nursing. *ViewPoint, 26*(4), 1, 8-12.

Hastings, C. (2006). The ambulatory care practice arena. In C.B. Laughlin (Ed.), *Core curriculum for ambulatory care nursing* (pp. 15-25). Pitman, NJ: American Academy of Ambulatory Care Nursing.

Joint Commission on Accreditation of Healthcare Organizations, The (JCAHO). (2004). *Assessing and improving staff competence* (CD-ROM). Oakbrook Terrace, IL: Joint Commission Resources.

Laughlin, C.B. (Ed.). (2006). *Core curriculum for ambulatory care nursing* (2nd ed.). Pitman, NJ: American Academy of Ambulatory Care Nursing.

Marcum, E.H., & West, R.D. (2004). Structured orientation for new graduates: A retention strategy. *Journal for Nursing Staff Development, 20*(3), 118-124.

McConnell, E. (1998). Competence and competency: Keeping your skills sharp. *Nursing 1998.*

Swan, B.A. (2007). Transitioning from acute care to ambulatory care. *Nursing Economic$, 25*(2), 130-134.

Additional Readings

Connelley, L.M., & Hoffart, N. (1998). A research-based model of nursing orientation. *Journal of Nursing Staff Development, 14*(1), 31-39.

Joint Commission, The. (2008). *Standards for ambulatory care.* Oakbrook Terrace, IL: Joint Commission Resources.

McKeown, E. (2003). Orienting new nurses. *ViewPoint, 25*(2), 10-12.

Chapter 2

STAFF ORIENTATION AND COMPETENCY PROGRAM CONTENT

Organizational/Systems Role of the Ambulatory Care Nurse

Lenora J. Flint, MSN, MS, RN, PHN, CNS
DiAnn Hughes, BA, ABRM

Healthcare economics, technology, research, evidence-based decision-making, and patient complexity have altered the roles and responsibilities of today's ambulatory care nurses. In response to these challenges, RNs must continually seek opportunities to enhance their knowledge for state of the art and safe nursing care competencies that employers and organizations seek. The future of health care reform and the nation's needs distinctly align with professional nursing. It is paramount to measure and communicate the RN's role and value in ambulatory care organizations.

Kitty Shulman, 2009 AAACN President, in her May/June 2009 AAACN *ViewPoint* article, "From the President: Articulating the Value of Nursing," indicated surprise in receiving survey comments from nurses needing help to articulate their value to their managers and administrators. These comments correlate with a perception that the role of the RN in primary care is diminishing and not valued. As a cost-saving measure, organizations are increasingly employing Medical Assistants (MAs) and Licensed Vocational Nurses (LVNs) rather than RNs. Additionally, some primary care clinics are experiencing high turnover of RNs who have expressed inability to use the full compliment of their "nursing expertise." It remains evident that RNs continue to perform a high volume of clerical tasks, such as message taking and appointment booking. This is a compromise of their appropriate healthcare delivery role, affecting their ability to provide direct support to physicians, direct patient care, and provide oversight of nursing functions. These ambulatory care trends contribute to RNs' inability to articulate their value.

In reality, the ambulatory care RN is a value-added member of the primary care team. Kitty Shulman (2009) provided data from the national Gallop and Harris polls that rank nurses as the most trustworthy professionals in America most recently for 2008. Furthermore, Unruh (2008) demonstrated that having more nurses on staff saves money. Childers (2008) indicated patient satisfaction scores are increasingly being linked to nursing care with several studies demonstrating a positive correlation between patients' perception of nursing care and their overall satisfaction with care provided. In today's tenuous environment, patient satisfaction is a hallmark of organizational viability.

The Organizational/Systems Role in which the RN practices is a defined healthcare structure encased with processes and resources purposefully designed to guide, support, and enable ambulatory nurses. This chapter promotes critical thinking, technical, and interpersonal skills in providing quality for ambulatory care patients. Competent staff is requisite for achieving quality care services; however, quality patient care services are equally dependent on the soundness of an organization's delivery systems and environmental supports.

Merriam-Webster (1994) describes an organization as the act or process of organizing or being organized; an administrative and functional structure characterized by complete conformity to the standards and requirements; it involves systematic planning and a united effort.

Similarly, a system is defined as a network of structures and channels; a function; related group of elements; a harmonious, orderly interaction. The application of these definitions is important on two levels. First, unmet goals often occur when organizations fail to define their structure and the significance of individual performance. Secondly, nurses may fail to understand they are a function within the system. Failure to understand and address these critical definitions may contribute to less than optimal outcomes for the organization and nursing. When nurses fail to embrace and own these definitions, quality, teamwork, and the reputation of nursing is adversely affected.

Ambulatory care nursing services encompass organized and systematic methodologies to assist patients in promoting wellness, preventing illness, and managing acute and chronic disease to affect the most attainable positive health status, over the life span (AAACN, 2005). Ambulatory care nursing is based on a philosophy committed to the delivery of efficient, cost-effective, and quality nursing care. Ambulatory care nurses practice within the organization/systems role when they manage and coordinate resources and workflow in their setting to assure a safe, comfortable, and hazard-free therapeutic environment for their patients, visitors, and colleagues.

It is paramount that RNs understand the metrics that substantiate their value and engage evidence-based nursing practice for clinical practice and organizational decision-making. Swan, Conway-Philips, and

Griffin (2006) specify the RN's value must be clearly delineated and identifiable, actionable, and quantifiable. Value exists as a part of an entire organization and not in isolation. Roberts (2007) indicated nurses can enhance their self-esteem and deepen their professional bonds with nurse colleagues by re-evaluating their roles and contributions to patient care. Communication steps to help this process include:

- Expressing pride in being a nurse
- Accepting and celebrating compliments about good patient care
- Actively complimenting others for work well done
- Looking for and acknowledging improvements to the system
- Being an ambassador to those outside the profession about the true contribution that nurses make to quality patient care

Significant challenges are experienced by ambulatory care RNs in today's complex organizational system. With the patient as the central focus, effective RNs understand their patient/nursing advocacy role and the organization's healthcare continuum structure. The scenarios in this chapter are reality-based and identify RN skills and behaviors that promote advocacy. The examples are designed to promote optimal performance, competent care, and nursing excellence. RNs that practice within this model can increase their visibility and the value of their actions on patient and organizational outcomes.

Follow Jill Jones, RN, as she meets everyday challenges in the ambulatory healthcare continuum. We encourage you to identify the professional nursing attributes Jill engages in her advocacy for patients and the nursing profession. *Key Action Tips* will help you to explore and apply these nursing characteristics.

---

1. **Dimension**: Practice/Office Support

   Definition:
   Practice office support in the ambulatory care setting is the delivery systems, environmental supports, as well as the competence and capability of the health care team.

   Introduction:
   Practice/office support is driven by key characteristics, including the organization's mission, patient demographics, and specialty practice. Ambulatory care organizations must consider their geographic location, for example, rural versus metro, and the level and quantity of available resources. Available resources are linked to geographic locations.

   Key Action Tips:
   - RNs understand principles that effectively contribute to a safe, accessible, and functional practice environment including the provision of appropriate supplies and equipment.
   - Establishment of metrics, ongoing monitoring, and process improvement of the practice environment is integral to the RN role.
   - RNs must articulate their economic cost savings.
   - Effective systems directly contribute to the organization's financial viability.
   - Leadership and learning are indispensable to each other.
   - Leadership is to influence, and is not limited to people in positions of authority.

   Example: Management of Equipment and Supplies
   - **Problem**
     The manager of the outpatient ambulatory care center has requested suggestions from staff to decrease the loss of surgical equipment which continues to be economically prohibitive to continue to replace. Additionally, physician complaints continue to escalate regarding their inability to provide surgical procedures timely and proficiently due to inadequate or missing equipment. Jill, a lead RN on the unit with the greatest equipment loss, shares the problem with her unit-based team (UBT), a multidisciplinary task force, including physician representation, created to improve patient outcomes. Led by Jill, who is currently serving as the chairperson of the UBT, they unanimously decide to tackle the problem.

   - **Solution**
     Using "mosquitoes" as a surgical equipment case in point, Jill and UBT colleagues map out each step the "mosquitoes" pass through to and from sterilization. They discover several gaps in the overall process, including lack of an ongoing tracking system to account for return of surgical equipment. Jill and the UBT document their process and develop a template to account for return of sterilized surgical equipment. Jill develops a PowerPoint presentation and shares the team's findings and recommendations including projected cost savings with the department manager who approves initiating the tracking system.

   - **Outcome**
     Reduction in cost expenditures for surgical equipment and assurance of availability of equipment for procedures accompanied by a cessation of physician complaints.

Subtopic	Elements	Competency Statement
Scheduling	➤ Scheduling types ➤ Provider variables ➤ Patient variables ➤ Support variables ➤ Scheduling system features and qualities ➤ No shows, cancellations, late arrivals, walk-ins, add-ons, sicker patients, and emergencies	Comprehends the intricacies of the member scheduling system and assures systems and resources support work volume and workflow.
Facility Planning and Space Utilization	➤ Location ➤ Layout and design	Evaluates and modifies facility planning and space utilization to enhance productivity and quality of care.
Environmental Management	➤ Safety ➤ Security ➤ Medical emergencies ➤ Infection control ➤ Emergency preparedness	Develops and engages ongoing monitoring and staff and member education to assure environmental management plans provide a safe, accessible, effective, and functional environment of care.
Management of Equipment and Supplies	➤ Medical equipment and supply selection ➤ Ordering/purchasing of equipment and supplies ➤ Inventory control ➤ Staff orientation/ongoing education and competency validation ➤ Ongoing assessment and monitoring ➤ Storage and recycling	Establishes and maintains medical equipment and supplies including a plan to promote safe and effective use of equipment.

2. **Dimension: Healthcare Fiscal Management**

Definition:
Healthcare fiscal management considers the origin of revenue and how actions and decisions affect resource management, program planning, and budget management.

Introduction:
In the current economic environment where hospitals and clinics are folding, new challenges abound for healthcare organizations and the populations they serve. Professional nurses must be conscious of how their clinical behaviors, at the point of care, impact revenue. Nurses must understand key monitors that affect revenue (e.g., emergency room visits, hospitalizations). The essence of ambulatory care work is health prevention and maintenance, which can reduce negative clinical outcomes. Preventative services may offset the costs of more extensive healthcare. Routine screening, such as mammography and pap tests, prevent manifestation of disease. The professional nurse understands and engages daily clinical behaviors to ensure quality patient care and fiscal solvency. You cannot talk quality without talking about cost.

Key Action Tips:
- Escalating cost increases the RN's role and responsibility in control and accountability.
- Health maintenance and preventive care processes promote fiscal solvency.
- RNs impact the cost/benefit ratio at the point of care.
- RNs are knowledgeable of disease management and how they can contribute to their operational component.

2. Dimension: Healthcare Fiscal Management (continued)

Example: Managed Care Concept

- **Problem**

  Ms. Harper presents to a nurse-run clinic for reading of her TB skin test. A routine part of patient appointments is a review of regular preventative health maintenance interventions. During the appointment, Jill, RN, determines per the electronic medical record, Ms. Harper is overdue to complete her preventative mammography.

- **Solution**

  Jill counsels Ms. Harper on the significance of a mammogram, provides her with education material, and assists her in scheduling the test prior to leaving the clinic. Jill also initiates communication to assure Ms. Harper receives an appointment reminder, consisting of a post-card and automated telephone message.

- **Outcome**

  Ms. Harper keeps her mammogram appointment. She is diagnosed with breast cancer, but due to early detection, her breast cancer is successfully treated. Jill enlists Ms. Harper to partner with the clinic team in presenting preventative health awareness programs to the community. Ms. Harper engages her personal experience with the mammogram as a practical example.

Subtopic	Elements	Competency Statement
Financial Environment of Health Care Organizations Revenue Sources Managed Care Concepts Coding Budget	➤ Access to care ➤ Plan of care ➤ Patient and/or family education ➤ Care/disease management ➤ Outcome measures	Applies knowledge of, financial principles, and resources to ensure that quality and appropriate care services are delivered in a cost-effective manner.

3. Dimension: Collaboration/Conflict Management

Definition:
Conflict is a situation in which two or more individuals have discordant perceptions and viewpoints impeding their ability to come to a mutual and shared resolution.

Introduction:
Conflict happens. However, conflict resolution takes courage and a strong resolve. Rather than view conflict as a negative experience, one can step back and view the differing experiences as an opportunity to strengthen relationships and identify common interests and outcomes while establishing a forum to more quickly resolve future challenges. RNs must be knowledgeable of behaviors that get in the way of conflict resolution, for example, avoidance, judging, accommodating, and blaming. These behaviors result in missed opportunities for patient advocacy, improved quality, and enhancement of self and professional worth.

Key Action Tips:
- Conflict is not always detrimental; conflict is a component of the "change process," and can generate innovation, creativity, increased efficiency, and improved outcomes.
- Daily, the RN is called upon to be a strong advocate for quality patient care and services. There is no substitute for professional confrontation. Not to do so can be seen as a sign of weakness.
- Speak the truth. Keeping silent or compromising one's integrity diminishes one's authentic self and increases dissatisfaction with the ambulatory care profession environment and how other healthcare groups perceive ambulatory care.
- Professional RNs search for common interest, do not personalize the conflict, and are courteous and respectful in acknowledging that everyone wants to do the right thing.

3. **Dimension: Collaboration/Conflict Management (continued)**

Example: Conflict Management
- **Problem**
Following her assessment and clinical interventions for Mr. Red's c/o of severe indigestion, Dr. Lamb initiates an IV and cardiac monitoring, placing him in the "holding area" awaiting test results. Dr. Lamb assigns her Unlicensed Assistant Personnel (UAP), Pat, to observe the patient.
- **Solution**
Jill, the rounding clinic RN, becomes aware of the UAP's assignment and immediately assumes responsibility for 1:1 patient monitoring for Mr. Red. The UAP becomes upset and complains to Dr. Lamb. Following Mr. Red's disposition by ambulance to the local hospital, Jill initiates a meeting with Dr. Lamb and Pat. Aware of impending conflict, Jill gathers UAP job description, competencies, and supportive facility policies and procedures. At the beginning of the meeting Jill shares the purpose for the meeting and proposed outcomes. Additionally, she collaborates with Pat and Dr. Lamb to identify basic resolution ground rules, for example, protecting each individual's self-respect, "no blame" approach, all participants have an equal voice and communication time for all participants, active listening, etc. The gathered supportive material is utilized to supplant Jill's contribution to resolving the conflict in an impartial manner.
- **Outcome**
All participants are educated regarding UAP boundaries while gaining appreciation of the UAP scope of work. Patient safety is assured by having the right health care discipline managing patients. Dr. Lamb's and Pat's attitude, understanding, and value of Jill as an RN and team leader is further enhanced. Jill experiences an increase in proactive consultation with her regarding department operations and patient care decisions by Dr. Lamb and Pat following the successful meeting outcomes.

Subtopic	Elements	Competency Statement
Collaboration	➤ Mission, vision, goals, and values ➤ Team norms ➤ Defined roles and responsibilities ➤ Delineated task with time lines ➤ Performance improvement monitors ➤ Open and honest communication ➤ Conflict management strategies ➤ A unified front: mutual trust, respect, and support ➤ Acknowledgement and value of diversity in style and scope-of-practice ➤ Shared responsibility and accountability ➤ Financial performance ➤ Data measures, reports, and analytical processes	Employs critical attributes of effective collaboration to create, promote, and maintain an environment that supports successful partnership and high performance team outcomes.
Conflict Management	➤ Communication styles ➤ Group dynamics ➤ Team problem-solving techniques ➤ Conflict management ➤ Constructive feedback modalities ➤ Cultural competency	Role models effective conflict resolution techniques with individuals and groups.

4. Dimension: Nursing Informatics

Definition:
Nursing informatics is a specialty that integrates nursing, computer, and information science to manage and communicate data, information, and knowledge in nursing practice (American Nurses Association [ANA], 2008).

Introduction:
Today's abundant technology supports ambulatory nurses' ability to apply informatics in clinical practice, administration, education, and research. Automated patient medical records serve as the central repository of data from other systems, for example, radiology, pharmacy, and laboratory. Many automated patient records link with national and international institutional data and registries. Decision support tools enhance the nurse's ability to make effective and timely decisions. The nurse must have ongoing knowledge and understanding, and must comply with standards of regulatory agencies specific to patient privacy and confidentiality.

Key Action Tips:
- RNs must be knowledgeable about and contribute to the information science dimensions of nursing and the organization.
- RNs must be knowledgeable of how to access informatics resources and to translate and evaluate findings to promote improved patient care and ambulatory nursing practice.
- RNs must be knowledgeable of how their clinical documentation impacts billing information and thus organizational viability.
- A patient's medical record can only be accessed in the delivery of patient care and/or a business need.

Example: Privacy and Confidentiality
- **Problem**
  While in town delivering a speech, George Clooney trips and hurts his ankle. He is taken to "urgent care" located within a local ambulatory care facility for treatment. Word swiftly moves through the clinic that George Clooney is a patient and everyone is interested in getting a peek at him and his entourage. Additionally, staff begins telephoning family members and friends about the event. Following the actor's course of care, he is discharged from urgent care and returns to Hollywood. The next day, Jill, the urgent care RN who was on duty during delivery of medical care to Mr. Clooney, notices local newspapers have information about his personal health record that could only have come from someone who had access to the electronic medical record.
- **Solution**
  Suspecting a potential breach of confidentiality per policy and procedure, Jill immediately notifies the clinic administrator and compliance officer. Together they develop a rapid cycle plan to determine if a breach of privacy and confidentiality has occurred which could negatively impact the organization. The outcome of the investigation determines violations exist.
- **Outcome**
  The administrator and compliance officer immediately communicate the confidentiality and privacy policies to the entire staff, requiring everyone complete compliance training. Jill and an HR representative conduct 1:1 meetings with Urgent Care Personnel and initiate appropriate disciplinary action with those associated with the breach. Jill also recommends and assumes the lead role to develop a letter of apology to Mr. Clooney, outlining the steps urgent care and the clinic have taken to safeguard personal health information of patients. Jill's swiftness in notifying and working to abate further problems surrounding the event is formally acknowledged by administration. She also receives a personal letter of thanks from Mr. Clooney.

Subtopic	Elements	Competency Statement
Nursing Informatics and Applications	➤ Operating mechanism and function ➤ Assets and limitations ➤ Troubleshooting ➤ Resources ➤ Downtime procedures	Evaluates and translates processes/data provided by systems to promote improved patient care and organizational services, including the selection of future informatics systems and applications.

Subtopic	Elements	Competency Statement
Patient Record	➤ Decision support systems ➤ Minimum data set ➤ Nursing process ➤ Documentation strategies ➤ Continuity of care ➤ Data retrieval ➤ Legality	Applies knowledge of informatics technology to facilitate patient care services.
Privacy and Confidentiality	➤ Health Insurance Portability and Accountability Act (HIPAA) ➤ Systems protecting: • Unauthorized access and harm to patient care data (system security) • Accidental or intentional disclosure to unauthorized person or unauthorized data alteration (data security)	Practice safeguards patient health care data.

5. **Dimension: Context of Care Delivery/Models**

Definition:
Care practice predicated on evidence-based practice, the nursing process, and professional practice standards.

Introduction:
Care/case management is a widely-used approach to health care delivery in ambulatory care. Care coordination functions on a broader spectrum. The organization defines the care coordination framework which at minimum should include the vision, communication plan, quality improvement program, standards, and the multidisciplinary team. On the other hand, case management coordinates care of the individual patient or population.

Key Action Tips:
- The RN provides evidence-based, clinically competent care.
- The RN demonstrates critical thinking, reflection, and problem-solving.
- The RN assumes accountability for quality of care and health care outcomes.
- The RN contributes to continuous improvement of the ambulatory health care system.
- The RN accesses resources within the organizational framework to promote optimal care coordination.

Example: A Model for Care Delivery
- **Problem**
  The heart failure hospital readmission rate exceeds community standards.
- **Solution**
  Evidence-based research indicates utilization of a transitional care program (TCP) across the continuum of care serves to decrease heart failure readmissions. The components of TCP include early hospital identification of heart failure patients, compliance with Joint Commission core measures, and discharge home health referral. Home health visit should be within 48 hours of discharge, with a focused medication and treatment plan review. Lastly, it also includes ongoing follow-up by ambulatory heart failure care managers.
- **Outcome**
  Heart failure readmission rates meet community standards while exhibiting a personalized care experience for patients.

Subtopic	Elements	Competency Statement
Ambulatory Care	➤ Nursing care delivery model; access to care, direct intervention, care coordination ➤ Nursing process ➤ Ambulatory care nursing administration and practice standards ➤ Evidence-based practice/care	Nursing practice and decision-making is guided by a conscientious use of theory and research.

6. Dimension: Care of the Caregiver

Definition:
"Someone whose life is in some way restricted by the need to be responsible for the care of someone who is mentally ill, mentally handicapped, physically disabled or whose health is impaired by sickness or old age" (Pitkeathley, 1989).

Introduction:
The number of caregivers in the workforce has increased threefold in the last five years and will continue to increase in the next ten years. Guilt is a common feeling in the landscape of care giving. When we take on the responsibility of caring for a loved one, we expect our lives to change. What is unexpected, and often goes unnoticed, is the forfeiting of our own well-being in order to become a primary caregiver. Stress associated with unsupported care for chronically ill family members may result in a condition commonly referred to as *caregiver syndrome*.

Key Action Tips:
- The RN provides care to the patient and family/significant other.
- The RN is knowledgeable of caregiver assets and challenges.
- The RN is caregiver-friendly; he or she designs and provides services and identifies resources with the needs of the caregiver in mind.

Example: Care of the Caregiver
- **Problem**
  For the past 3 months, Jean has been traveling between California and Pennsylvania to take care of her elderly father who has served as the primary caregiver for his wife. Recently Jean's father was hospitalized for cancer. Jean's cousin is temporarily helping with the care of her parents until she arrives from California. Following Jean's arrival, her father is discharged from the hospital and scheduled for outpatient chemotherapy sessions. During a chemotherapy treatment, Jill, the clinic RN, finds Jean crying in the waiting room.
- **Solution**
  Morally and ethically bound, Jill takes Jean privately aside to assess the situation. Jean shares her concerns and fears about her parents and questions her ability to continue to provide adequate support for them. Jean feels overwhelmed and helpless from everything that is going on.
- **Outcome**
  Following the discussion, Jill initiates a team conference to develop a plan of care for Jean and her parents. The team conference includes the oncologist and primary care physician, social service, and the nursing chemotherapy staff. Jean is provided with local resources including support groups, community resources, and a direct telephone number to maintain linkage with staff following her return to California. Jean vocalizes her appreciation and feelings of comfort to Jill and the clinic team.

Subtopic	Elements	Competency Statement
Caregiver	➤ Partnership/team member ➤ Plan of care ➤ Education ➤ Internal and external resources ➤ Respite ➤ Terminally ill	RN organizes and plans for the special needs of caregivers throughout a patient's disease trajectory.

7. **Dimension: Priority Management/Delegation and Supervision**

Definition:
Priority management is the ability to manage and direct patient access and flow for effective and efficient clinical operations (Weinstein, 2004).
Delegation is the transfer of responsibilities for the performance of a task from one (competent) person to another (American Nurses Association [ANA], 1997).
Supervision is the direction and oversight of the performance of others (Laughlin, 2006, p. 425).

Introduction:
The RN provides oversight and is accountable for efficient and effective operations within the ambulatory care environment. This responsibility requires RNs to have a detailed understanding of the purpose, goals, and objectives of the care delivery system in which they work and their requisite authority. The care delivery system, for example, urgent care, pediatrics, and OB/GYN differ; each setting requires priority management of patients and interventions, staff mix, skill set and competencies, supplies, and resources to maximize clinic operations and patient outcomes. The RN assures patients receive the *right* level of care, in the *right* setting, at the *right* time, by the *right* caregiver using the *right* equipment and supplies and who has the *right* supervision.

Key Action Tips:
- RNs supervise others.
- No one works under the RN's license except the licensee.
- The RN engages staff competencies in the work setting when delegating tasks.
- The RN executes the 3 key stages of supervision: communication, level of required oversight, and outcomes evaluation.
- The RN is knowledgeable of one's nurse practice act and policies specific to delegation and supervision.

Example: Delegation and Supervision
- **Problem**
  Jill, a new RN supervisor, identifies a high RN turnover and that RNs in the primary care clinic are assigned to message management and are not involved in the coordination and direct management of patient care activities. Further investigation reveals the majority of messages are clerical, for example, appointment booking, requests to have physician telephone patient, etc. The clinic manages a high volume of patients with respiratory problems with physicians handing off patients to UAPs and LVNs for breathing treatments. The patients are discharged by the UAPs and/or LVNs upon conclusion of treatment.
- **Solution**
  Jill conducts a gap analysis and develops a PowerPoint presentation to share outcomes and goals with staff and physicians. An ad hoc task force led by Jill develops workflow processes to reposition staff, specifically RNs, based upon their scope of practice/work. Following review of everyone's scope of practice/work, clerical work previously managed by RNs is redirected to the UAPs and LVNs. Clinic RNs assume the responsibility for breathing treatments and assessment of discharge readiness of patients and other tasks befitting their role.
- **Outcome**
  Jill repositions staff based upon their scope of practice/work. These changes ensure patient safety and improve RN morale. Jill forecasts a decrease in RN turnover which she will continue to track.

Subtopic	Elements	Competency Statement
Priority Management	➤ Rapid and efficient triage ➤ Appropriate care at the appropriate level; right access, time frame, providers, care and follow-up ➤ RN interventions focused on patients with complex and emergent nursing needs	Directs the flow of patients and staff to assure patients are adequately managed, and the clinic runs smoothly and effectively.
Delegation and Supervision	➤ Patient care and work performance standards ➤ Professional practice standards, role expectation, and level of competency ➤ Right task assigned to the right person ➤ RN proprietary of patient assessment and coordination of care ➤ Delegated task supported by clear, concise descriptions with expected task outcomes, timelines and resources ➤ Supervision and evaluation of the progress of assigned task and outcomes ➤ Staff feedback; respectful, constructive, and non-confrontational	Directs and guides the performance outcomes of RNs, LPN/LVNs, and UAPs as manifested in the state practice act/ guidelines and the institution's job descriptions. Practice embodies legal responsibilities and delegation, supervision, and communication principles.

8. Dimension: Multicultural Nursing Care in the Ambulatory Care Setting

Definition:
Multicultural nursing care recognizes the cultural values and beliefs individuals and groups bring to the health care setting.

Introduction:
Ambulatory nursing care occurs within a multicultural environment. RNs need an understanding of cultural beliefs and practices to effectively plan and provide culturally competent care. Culture and beliefs impact prevention, health maintenance, and self-care management. References describe three components of multicultural health care delivery and indicate care should be culturally sensitive, culturally appropriate, and culturally competent (Spector, 2004). It is unrealistic for RNs to become competent with all cultural groups; however, learning about predominant cultural groups in the geographic area in which they practice is paramount.

Key Action Tips:
- Providing culturally competent healthcare is a professional and social mandate in modern healthcare.
- The RN must explore one's own cultural background, values, and beliefs – especially related to health and healthcare.
- The RN must examine one's own cultural biases towards people whose culture differs from one's own culture.

Example: Multicultural Needs
- **Problem**
  Clinic data reflects an increase in the diabetic population during the past three years. Analysis of the data identifies an increase in the Hispanic diabetic population. A major component of treatment for diabetes is healthy diet. Current education materials do not include healthy approaches to preparing foods common to Hispanics.

8. Dimension: Multicultural Nursing Care in the Ambulatory Care Setting (continued)

- **Solution**
  Conduct a literature search for evidence-based practice, for example from the American Diabetes Association. Collaborate with the local health education and dietary departments and Hispanic community resources. Identify competent interpreter resources (internal and external) to assist in delivering the dietary information in Spanish. Develop and use education material at 4th to 6th grade reading level.
- **Outcome**
  Program assessment by participants indicates favorable responses and expressed appreciation for development of dietary educational program supportive of the Hispanic culture and lifestyle. For those who attended the program, the data continues to demonstrate an improvement in HgA1C versus the Hispanic diabetes population who did not attend the program.

Subtopic	Elements	Competency Statement
Culturally Competent Care	➤ Cultural diversity knowledge and intervention techniques ➤ Cultural learning environment ➤ Mutual trust and respect for differences among individuals and groups ➤ Acknowledgment of the contributions of each individual ➤ Valued and integrated cultural variations	Utilizes expertise in cultural competency to enhance relationships, processes, and outcomes for consumers and providers.

9. Dimension: Ongoing Political/Entrepreneurial Skills

Definition: Entrepreneur
An RN who has assumes responsibility to advocate and promote ambulatory nursing practice and healthcare. The individual and collective voice of nursing is paramount to influencing political healthcare policy and reform.

Introduction:
The RN is resolute in support of ambulatory care nursing as a specialty and professional entity. Ambulatory care offers diverse entrepreneurial opportunities, for example leading or participating in clinical and healthcare systems research to improve health care and organizational effectiveness. Such efforts identify ambulatory care practice as essential to the continuum of accessible, high quality, and cost-effective health care (AAACN Identity Statement). Florence Nightingale was an exemplary role model in reforming healthcare at the local, national, and international level.

Key Action Tips:
- Maintain ongoing and active membership with professional and specialty nursing organizations.
- Serve on ethics, educational, quality, and other workplace committees.
- Subscribe to nursing journals and review current nursing practice literature.
- Initiate and implement innovative practices and concepts.
- Understand relevant legislation and the impact on local and national ambulatory care practice.

9. **Dimension: Ongoing Political/Entrepreneurial Skills (continued)**

Example: Business Endeavors
- **Problem**
Jill, a newly hired experienced staff RN, joins a primary care clinic. In her previous employment as a staff nurse, Jill was a team leader, actively involved in supervising staff and the workflow of the department to assure effective clinic processes. During her first few months, Jill finds RNs are not fully engaged in leading and directing patient care activities, resulting in decisions by LVNs and UAPs beyond their scope of practice/work. The physicians are complaining of staff performance problems and the inability to meet department goals.
- **Solution**
Jill approaches the new Director to share her observations and the physicians' concerns. Central to her observations is the RNs' failure to supervise and provide oversight for the LVNs and UAPs. Jill shares information on nursing leadership gleaned from the literature and suggests pulling together a task force to ensure appropriate RN leadership. Given her past experience and literature review, she presents a draft proposal for an RN leadership program. A task force consisting of the staff educator, Director, and RN, LVN, UAP representatives begins by reviewing the proposal and literature. The Director guides them through a cause and effect analysis, resulting in acceptance of the proposal with minor modifications.
- **Outcome**
Program outcome metrics are developed and the program is administered by the staff education department. RN attendance at the program is mandatory and occurs over the next six months. After three months, RN team leaders are assigned staff. Under the new process, staff is appropriately directing nursing clinical practice issues to the RNs rather than the physicians and director. Ongoing metrics are beginning to shift favorably including physician and patient satisfaction.

Subtopic	Elements	Competency Statement
Professional Organizations	➤ Professional membership ➤ Continuing education ➤ Professional standards of care ➤ Clinical practice guidelines ➤ Literature review ➤ Nursing research ➤ Facility and public policy development ➤ Lobbying efforts ➤ Consultant	Participates and contributes to internal and external committees and professional organizations.
Business Endeavors	➤ Corporate compliance standards ➤ Quality indicators ➤ Internal and external regulatory processes ➤ Clinical initiatives	Engages knowledge of health care, philosophy, mission, goals, objectives, and business plan to bridge patient care services and outcomes.

10. **Dimension: Structuring Customer-Focused Systems**

Definition: Customer Service
According to Turban et al. (2002), "Customer service is a series of activities designed to enhance the level of customer satisfaction – that is, the feeling that a product or service has met the customer expectation." Customer service may be provided by a person (e.g., RN, receptionist, MD, billing office, pharmacy lab, etc.), or by automated means called *self-service*. Examples of self-service are Internet sites, registration kiosks, automated appointment reminder phone calls, etc.

10. Dimension: Structuring Customer-Focused Systems (continued)

Introduction:
In the past, the healthcare industry has not always had a central focus on service and creating an optimal patient care experience. The healthcare mentality was "the patient needs us or is dependent upon us." Today we have an abundance of healthcare providers with a wide range of expertise resulting in a variety of choices with providers and healthcare organizations competing for the same patients. Savvy patients today have access to report cards identifying outcomes to compare the quality and costs of care. With increased competition the market has shifted; premier healthcare service and quality now means survival. A major component of healthcare risk management mitigation is customer service. Historical studies demonstrate patients in the aggregate sue as a result of impolite healthcare staff rather than for clinical reasons. Organizations can use service to retain and grow their business.

Key Action Tips:
- The RN demonstrates the 3 levels of caring: competence (what we do), courtesy (what we say), and compassion (what we feel).
- The RN provides compassion – the unique service in healthcare.
- The RN uses flexibility to focus on courtesy and compassion to supersede efficiency.
- The RN understands satisfied patients pass positive care experiences about the organization to others.

Example: Customer Service
- **Problem**

  Ms. Smith, a very obese patient, comes regularly into the ambulatory HTN clinic for blood pressure checks. In spite of having extra large cuffs, it is sometimes difficult to obtain the patient's blood pressure because of her weight. Rebecca, a new RN, is assigned to the clinic for the day and struggles to obtain a blood pressure reading on Ms. Smith. Jill, the RN preceptor, overhears Rebecca tell the patient, "This would not be so difficult if you would lose some weight. No wonder you are hypertensive. If you would lose about 75 pounds, your blood pressure would be in control." Ms. Smith begins to cry uncontrollably as she has lost 50 pounds over the past year in a weight management program and her blood pressure continues to improve because of her weight loss.

- **Solution**

  Jill immediately intervenes and directs Rebecca to wait for her at the nurses' station. Jill apologizes to Ms. Smith for the Rebecca's behavior while comforting the patient. Jill is familiar with Ms. Smith, a volunteer coordinator in the community. Jill reviews Ms. Smith's medical history with emphasis on the improvement in her health that she has achieved, encouraging her to continue. Jill takes her blood pressure, which is normal; her weight is down another 4 pounds. Ms. Smith and Jill are delighted with today's outcomes. Jill assesses Ms. Smith's emotions, which are positive. They spend a few moments with social chatter and Jill ends the visit by scheduling Ms. Smith's return appointment.

- **Outcome**

  Following Ms. Smith's departure, Jill takes Rebecca to the conference room and asks her if she knows why the visit was interrupted. Rebecca replies, "I don't have a clue." Jill utilizes this opportunity to coach Rebecca regarding the organization's customer service standards which engage the three levels of caring: competency (what we do), courtesy (what we say), and compassion (what we feel). Members, patients, and their families are more likely to feel welcomed, cared for, and amenable to improve their health when they experience all levels of caring. While the comments Rebecca made were true, the words and her delivery were demeaning and demonstrated disregard for Ms. Smith. Rebecca expresses that her intent was to motivate; however, she now understands she offended Ms. Smith and states she will apologize to her during her next appointment.

Subtopic	Elements	Competency Statement
Customer Service	➤ Primary consumer concerns; access to healthcare, reasonable cost, quality services ➤ Customer service standards ➤ Patient Bill of Rights ➤ HIPAA ➤ Complaint resolution process ➤ Communication techniques ➤ Cultural competency	Treats every patient/family with dignity and worth; acknowledging their individuality and autonomy.

11. Dimension: Workplace Regulatory Compliance

Definition: Compliance
What we must do daily to maintain a good reputation and to comply with all applicable laws, regulations, and accreditation standards.

Introduction:
Today, health care organizations are under intense scrutiny by regulatory agencies and the public. Effective compliance standards foster a culture where conformity with State and Federal law and regulation is the accepted standard to promote excellent patient care. Organizations should evaluate the necessity of efforts that are cross-functional and integrated with established priorities for internal controls.

Key Action Tips:
- Each RN is responsible for doing his or her part to uphold compliance standards.
- The RN understands, articulates, and role models the organization's commitment to compliance and ethical and legal conduct.
- The RN looks for and speaks up about compliance standard improprieties.
- The RN speaks up and consults with compliance resources when unsure of what to do.
- RNs grant others the same respect and fair treatments they expect for themselves.

Example: Workplace Regulatory Compliance
- **Problem**

  Barbara, a home health RN, is assigned to manage 25 wound care patients Monday through Friday. One of her patients calls Jill, the RN supervisor, and states his wound care had not been provided yesterday. Jill assures the patient she will investigate and get back to him. Jill reviews the patient's medical record which indicates that wound care was provided. During Barbara's vacation, Regina assumes the management of her patients. Several patients express to Regina that they have not been provided with wound care on a regular basis and the dressings appear to be older than the time the medical records state wound care was completed. Regina is concerned and reports her findings to Jill.

- **Solution**

  Jill obtains and reviews all relevant medical records. The documentation reflects that wound care has been provided; however, she notices the documentation is identical for all patients regardless of their wound condition. Jill decides to conduct a survey of Barbara's patients to assess their perception of the organization's wound care services. Following her analysis of the patients' feedback, Jill concludes that wound care does not appear to have been provided as documented by Barbara. A meeting is established with Barbara and findings presented. Several concerns and disparities were shared with Barbara, including wound care services that were documented as provided to three patients on the same date and time. Following review of the information, Barbara confesses to her supervisor that she has not always been providing care to patients.

- **Outcome**

  Jill consults with the Human Resource Department and the compliance officer. They perform an investigation of the events and conclude Barbara has falsified the medical record, resulting in inaccurate coding, failed to follow physician orders and provide individualized patient care, inaccurate payroll reporting, and misrepresenting the organization. Barbara is terminated from the organization for these fraudulent acts and is reported to the state Board of Nursing.

Subtopic	Elements	Competency Statement
Workplace Regulatory Compliance	➤ Equal Employment Opportunity Commission (EEOC) ➤ Occupational Safety and Health Administration (OSHA)	Practice illustrates compliance with equal opportunity and workplace safety regulations.

12. Dimension: Advocacy (Inter-Organizational and Community)

Definition:
Advocacy is the act or process of advocating or supporting a cause or proposal on behalf of another.

Introduction:
Nurses are one of the most trusted health care professionals because of their historic track record of advocating on behalf of patients/families. The most effective nurse advocates have a passion for and a keen understanding of health/disease management and the healthcare delivery systems. Their knowledge is transferred to patients to promote self-care management and help the patient/family navigate a complex and ever-changing health system. Nurse advocates serve on key local and national health care decision-making committees.

Key Action Tips:
- Help patients/families understand their rights and responsibilities.
- Develop and role model astute communication and negotiation skills.
- Maintain membership in nursing organizations (such as AAACN).

Example: Inter-Organizational Advocacy
- **Problem**
  During these economic times, clinics are seeing more patients who have experienced a change in or loss of their health care benefits limiting their ability to continue health care services.
- **Solution**
  Jill, RN team leader, forms a task force of key stakeholders including physicians, social workers, administrators, pharmacists, community leaders, etc., to assess internal and external resources available to support patients and their families. The three most common needs identified by the task force for this population are transportation, medication, and food assistance.
- **Outcome**
  Internally, patients are "fast tracked" to onsite clinic financial counselors to help them apply for health care assistance programs. Establishment of a referral relationship with free community clinics, food banks, and free dollar ride transportation for health services.

Subtopic	Elements	Competency Statement
Inter-Organizational Advocacy	➤ Societal contract ➤ Access to care ➤ Nursing process ➤ Patient/family education ➤ Continuity of care ➤ Informed decision-making ➤ Patient satisfaction ➤ Ethics ➤ Organization/patient/family partnership ➤ Complaint resolution process ➤ Customer service ➤ Clinical practice standards ➤ Advance directives ➤ Performance improvement ➤ Discharge planning ➤ Cost containment ➤ Disease/population care management	Engages opportunities to act in the best interest of the patient/family, building trust and confidence, while upholding moral and legal standards of due care.

Subtopic	Elements	Competency Statement
Inter-Organizational Advocacy (continued)	➤ Patient self-determination act ➤ Cultural diversity ➤ Autonomy ➤ Discharge planning	Coordinates mechanisms across systems, institutions, and community to provide continuity of care.
Community Advocacy	➤ Community activities ➤ Professional organizations	Participates in community and professional activities to promote health education and a positive image of healthcare systems.

13. Dimension: Legal Issues

Definition:
Health care is bound by laws and regulations. When these are violated, it can lead to wide spectrum of legal issues that can impact patient/families, the health care team, and the organization's survival and image.

Introduction:
Health care organizations face an increased complexity of laws and greater scrutiny by outside agencies and patient advocacy groups. This creates a challenge for the ambulatory care nurse to maintain ongoing compliance. Given the circumstances, nurses must understand laws and standards relevant to their practice, while safeguarding patients and the organization. Ethical dilemmas may surface requiring consultation with healthcare risk management, leadership, and the bioethics committee. A major legal issue in health care is accurate and complete documentation. Liability may exist when the nurse does not use good documentation standards.

Key Action Tips:
- Each nurse is accountable for his or her practice and is not protected by the license of another practitioner.
- Adhere to elements of good documentation.
- An error is defined as an omission or co-omission.
- Error communication is important whether a patient is harmed or not; you cannot fix things unless you know the problem.

Example: Legal Issues
- **Problem**
  Jill, an experienced RN preceptor, is assigned to orient Stephanie, a new RN, to the clinic. Jill witnessed Stephanie drawing up a medication. Upon further questioning, Jill determines Stephanie has drawn up a "sound-a-like" medication; MD ordered Solu-Medrol IM, Stephanie retrieved Depo-Medrol IM. Fortunately an error was diverted. Jill immediately takes the opportunity to review medication administration principles with Stephanie including clinic policies and procedures. Over the next few weeks, Jill's concerns intensify as she continues to witness Stephanie's failure to adhere to the 5 rights of medication administration.
- **Solution**
  Jill meets with the clinic supervisor to review her documented concerns and data regarding Stephanie.
- **Outcome**
  Jill and her supervisor meet with Stephanie to determine how she feels she is doing overall including her medication administration performance. Jill's preceptor assessment of Stephanie's performance specific to medication administration is conveyed. Through this discussion, gaps in performance are identified and a mutual performance improvement plan is developed. Stephanie's preceptorship period is extended to assure patient safety standards are met. The group agrees on the frequency of follow-up meetings to review Stephanie's progress.

Subtopic	Elements	Competency Statement
Consent	➤ Informed consent; definition and components ➤ Patient self-determination act ➤ Exceptions to informed consent ➤ Legal competency ➤ Legal incompetence ➤ Persons/entities who may provide consent when one is deemed legally incompetent ➤ Tools and documentation standards	Interprets and applies legal knowledge of verbal and/or written consents, assuring standards are met.
Transfers	➤ Emergency Medical Treatment and Active Labor Act (EMTALA) ➤ Protected persons ➤ Transfer requirements ➤ Penalties and safeguards	Provides same level of care and management for all patients presenting at an emergency department regardless of ability to pay.
Abandonment	➤ Definition ➤ Liability ➤ Legal termination	Affirms advanced practice nurses provide care to patients until the patient-provider relationship is legally terminated.
Reportable Situations	➤ Facility and state reportable malpractice and/or quality situations ➤ Internal and external reporting structures and processes ➤ Nursing malpractice; elements of negligence ➤ Ethical dilemmas	Assumes responsibility for own actions and evokes an ethical obligation to report incompetent nursing practice.
Documentation	➤ Legal significance ➤ Best practice documentation standards ➤ Subject matter/content focus ➤ Computerized documentation and safety	Authored confirmation in the medical record reflects knowledge and adherence of documentation standards, serving as legal proof of the type and quality of nursing care provided to patients.
Telephone	➤ Facility protocol for telephone orders ➤ Documentation ➤ AAACN telephone practice standards and triage protocols	Practice behaviors safeguard against liability issues resulting from telephonic health care interactions.
Regulation of Nursing Practice	➤ Nurse Practice Act ➤ AAACN *Core Curriculum* (Laughlin, 2006) ➤ AAACN competencies ➤ Scope of practice for other disciplines	Practice is commensurate with the standards of the State Nursing Practice Act and the ambulatory care organization's delineated RN role, responsibilities, and competencies.

14. Dimension: Workload

Definition:
Workload is the volume and complexity of patient care needs and other related activities that nurses must timely achieve.

Introduction:
Evidence-based workload and staffing methodologies for ambulatory care are limited. Ambulatory care nursing is a specialty and cannot depend on inpatient nursing as a model for staffing and recruitment. Ambulatory care workload and staffing must be based upon ambulatory care specialty delivery characteristics. Patients are in the ambulatory care setting for a limited period of time and within that timeframe priorities are established to meet primary, secondary, and tertiary prevention. The RN must be conscious of the patient's reason for visit as well as his or her total health care needs, for example immunizations and cancer screens. The RN utilizes his or her leadership skills to guide the work of other nursing disciplines and unlicensed personnel to achieve aforementioned goals.

Key Action Tips:
- RNs understand the scope of practices for RNs, LVN/LPNs, and unlicensed assistant personnel (scope of work).
- RNs integrate the knowledge of the scheduling and decision support systems to develop care delivery for the day.

Example: Staffing and Skill Mix
- **Problem**
  The Pediatrics Clinic's medical assistant (MA) to nurse ratio is 3:1 and the clinic administers a high volume of immunizations. A primary responsibility of the medical assistant is immunization administration. Their medications must be reviewed by licensed personnel prior to administration. During the flu season 30% of the staff is out sick. Jill, the RN team leader, must ensure adequate licensed personnel are available to review all MA medications before administration.
- **Solution**
  Jill arrives early each morning to review sick calls and contacts the central staffing office for replacement personnel to assure provision of all clinic services including assignment of licensed personnel to each team for medication verification.
- **Outcome**
  Overall clinic services are maintained including immunizations.

Subtopic	Elements	Competency Statement
Staffing and Skill Mix	➤ Organization's mission, services, and standards of care ➤ Nursing care delivery model ➤ Environmental factors ➤ Staffing and skill mix ratio; protocol and tools ➤ Staff competencies ➤ Patient population care needs; patient intensity ➤ Patient scheduling process and planned procedures ➤ Environmental factors	Analyzes multiple variables to assure staff and skill mix ratio is sufficient to adequately serve the volume of patients and the complexity of their needs.

Subtopic	Elements	Competency Statement
Staff Recruitment and Retention	➤ Posting/advertisement/recruitment fairs ➤ Job description; minimum requirements ➤ Interview process ➤ Orientation plan and competency development	Contributes to retention and recruitment efforts by effective role modeling and participation in recruitment and retention processes.
Ambulatory Care Orientation	➤ Preceptor, coach, and/or competency validator ➤ Organizational and department culture, mission, goals, and objectives ➤ Collegial working relationships; professional work environment ➤ Reporting relationships and accountabilities ➤ Role expectations; ambulatory care nursing roles; clinical, organization/systems, and professional nursing ➤ Critical thinking, clinical/technical, and interpersonal domains of competency ➤ Equipment and procedures ➤ Organization, department, and community resources ➤ New employee satisfaction monitor	Utilizes a planned orientation program guided by measurable competency statements and tools to verify employee is capable of safe, independent performance.
Productivity Monitoring	➤ Strategic plans ➤ Cost of care ➤ Financial performance ➤ Patient, staff, and provider satisfaction ➤ Health status ➤ Complication incidence ➤ Access and availability ➤ "Report Card" measures and outcomes ➤ Volume visit ➤ Quality improvement; risk management ➤ Sentinel events	Employs varied outcome measures to analyze and enhance patient outcomes and staff/organization effectiveness.

15. Dimension: Competencies

Definition:
Competence means having the ability to demonstrate the technical, critical thinking, and interpersonal skills necessary to perform one's job responsibilities.

Introduction:
All nursing staff within ambulatory care must possess the appropriate skill and ability to meet the organization's standards. Nurses must undergo necessary and appropriate training to maintain their skills. Competency assessment is not an event, but an ongoing validation process in the clinical setting. Administrators of ambulatory care assure effective processes beginning with recruitment and hiring, and continuing with orientation and performance evaluation. A standard competency tool that clearly defines the critical elements of performance is used to guide the training and validation processes. AAACN has identified core competencies for ambulatory care RNs which can be used to structure competency validation.

Key Action Tips:
- Competency validation is not coaching; nurses must demonstrate that they can perform independently in their role and responsibilities.
- Validation is to occur in the clinical setting with patients and with a few exceptions (for example, a mock code blue), should not be a simulation.

Example: Competency Evaluation Process
- **Problem**
  Tilli has recently transferred to the ambulatory care department. She has 8 years of critical care nursing experience. Following her orientation, her competencies are validated in the clinical setting and she is challenged in performing telehealth assessments and her performance is rated as a novice. Tilli is vividly upset and contends that Jill, RN validator, has not rated her accurately. She verbalizes to Jill that she has historically been rated as expert at prior inpatient competency skill labs.
- **Solution**
  Jill meets with the manager and reviews Tilli's competency ratings and shares that she is not satisfied with the competency validation process. The manager reviews Jill's competency process and documentation to assure that her assessment was appropriate. Having experienced this before with other transferring inpatient nurses, she is comfortable with Jill's ratings. The manager and Jill develop a plan to review and reinforce with Tilli ambulatory care's philosophy and approach to competency validation.
- **Outcome**
  Following the discussion, Tilli vocalizes her understanding of validation conducted via a skill lab versus the clinical setting. They discuss the definition of *novice* and explain that she is new to the ambulatory setting and processes including telehealth assessments. Together they identify Tilli's barrier that she thought telephone assessment was different than a face-to-face assessment. The manager and Jill explain that 90% of an assessment is questions and the patient's response regardless of whether the patient is physically present or not. An improvement plan is developed to provide Tilli with AAACN telehealth standards and training. Through this process, Tilli gains knowledge and utilizes the reference tools. Within three months she independently performs telehealth assessments at a competent level.

Subtopic	Elements	Competency Statement
Competency Evaluation Process	➤ Hiring process ➤ Orientation ➤ Ongoing assessment and validation in the clinical setting ➤ Annual performance evaluation	Engages the full spectrum of competency evaluation at all stages.
Competency Domains	➤ Interpersonal skill ➤ Critical thinking skill ➤ Technical/psychomotor skill	Understands and applies the appropriate domain in evaluating competency.

Subtopic	Elements	Competency Statement
Competency Rating Levels	➤ Novice – Can undertake skill but must be supervised/checked by a validator. Completes skill elements but beyond time frames. Requires assistance from the appropriate persons. May need to review the policy/procedure but needs minimal prompting. ➤ Independent – Undertakes the skill easily, readily, with time frames, without any assistance or prompting. ➤ Expert – Can teach the skill and is a resource to others. Has in-depth understanding of the skill and problem-solving. Works at maximum level of efficiency and confidence. Functions as a trainer or validator in the department for the skill. ➤ Not-met – Cannot undertake the skill. Does not or is unable to perform the skill despite following policy/procedure or given assistance/prompting. Continues to make the same mistakes.	Utilizes the competency rating scale to document performance outcomes and support improvement plan development.
Performance Improvement Plan	➤ Individualized, role- or department-based ➤ Measurable outcomes ➤ Timeframe	Uses a performance improvement process to develop competency.
Education Plan	➤ High-volume/high-risk/problem-prone ➤ Solicit input from staff and physicians ➤ Considers organization's mission, vision, and values	Builds a plan that considers current and future department systems, processes, and outcomes.

References

American Academy of Ambulatory Care Nursing (AAACN). (2005). *A guide to ambulatory care nursing orientation and competency assessment.* Pitman, NJ: Author.

American Nurses Association (ANA). (1997). *Report of the ANA Council/NNSDO Taskforce on Advanced Practice Nursing, Continuing Education, and Staff Development.* Pensacola, FL: National Nursing Staff Development Organization.

American Nurses Association (ANA). (2008). *Scope and standards of practice for nursing professional development.* Washington, D.C.: Author.

Childers, L. (2008, May 5). Knowing the score. *NurseWeek (California),* 28-29.

Laughlin, C.B. (Ed.). (2006). *Core curriculum for ambulatory care nursing* (2nd ed.). Pitman, NJ: American Academy of Ambulatory Care Nursing.

Merriam-Webster's collegiate dictionary (10th ed.). (1994). Springfield, MA: Merriam-Webster.

Pitkeathley, B. (1989). *It's my duty, isn't it?* London: Souvenir Press.

Roberts, S.J. (2007, Feb/Mar). Colleagues, co-workers or enemies. *Nurses World Magazine,* 26-30.

Shulman, K. (2009). From the president: Articulating the value of nursing. *ViewPoint, 31*(3), 2, 13.

Spector, R.E. (2004). *Cultural diversity in health and illness* (6th ed.). Upper Saddle River, NJ: Pearson Education.

Swan, B., Conway-Phillips, R., & Griffin, K. (2006). Demonstrating the value of the RN in ambulatory care. *Nursing Economic$, 24*(6), 315-322.

Turban, E. (2002). *Electronic commerce: A managerial perspective* (2nd ed.). New Jersey: Prentice Hall.

Unruh, L. (2008). Nurse staffing and patient, nurse, and financial outcomes. *American Journal of Nursing, 108*(1), 62-71.

Weistein, S. (2004). Strategic partnerships: Bridging the collaboration gap. *Journal of Infusion Nursing, 27*(5), 297-301.

Additional Readings

American Academy of Ambulatory Care Nursing (AAACN). (2010). *Scope and standards of practice for professional ambulatory care nursing* (8th ed.) Pitman, NJ: Author.

Bensing, K. (2006, May). Collaboration in healthcare. *ADVANCE for Nurses,* 19-22.

Board of Registered Nursing. (2004). Nursing Practice Act: Rules and Regulations. Sacramento, CA.

Carroll, P. (2006). *Nursing leadership and management: A practical guide.* Clifton Park, NY: Thomson Delmar Learning.

Exstron, S. (2001). The state board of nursing and its role in continued competency. *The Journal of Continuing Education in Nursing, 32*(3), 118-125.

Griffin, K. (2009). Committed to continual learning. *ViewPoint, 31*(1), 2-11.

Hudson, T. (2008). Delegation: Building a foundation for our future nurse leaders. *MEDSURG Nursing, 17*(6), 396-421.

Kaiser Permanente Tricentral Staff Education Department. (2001). *Education framework and competency model.*

Kobbs, A. (1997). Questions and answers from the JCAHO: Competence: The shot heard around the nursing world. *Nursing Management, 28*(2), 10-13.

Laughlin, C.B. (2009). *Expert clinician role in ambulatory care nursing.* Presented May 14-15, 2009 at the Kaiser Permanente Ambulatory Nursing Symposium.

Lipe, S., & Beasely, S. (2004). *Critical thinking in nursing: A cognitive skills workbook.* Philadelphia: Lippincott Williams & Wilkins.

Paskche, S.M. (2009). *Nursing knowledge development in ambulatory care.* Presented May 14-15, 2009 at the Kaiser Permanente Ambulatory Nursing Symposium.

Restrepo, R.K. (2008, June 16). Who's in charge? *NurseWeek (California),* 14-15.

Samuel, M. (2006). *Creating the accountable organization: A practical guide to improve performance execution.* Katonah, NY: Xephor Press.

Schreiner, S., & Cote, J. (2009). Nursing education's role in optimizing the primary care nursing team in ambulatory setting. *ViewPoint, 31*(2), 1-11.

Tracy, J., & Summers, G. (2001). Competency assessment: A practical guide to the JCAHO standards. Marblehead, MA: Opus Communications, Inc.

Wright, D. (1998). *The ultimate guide to competency assessment in healthcare* (2nd ed.). Eau Claire, WI: Professional Education Systems, Inc.

Chapter 3

Clinical Nursing Practice Competencies, Office Visit

Carol Brautigam, MSN, RN
Linda Brixey, RN
Jane Hummer, BSN, MPH, RN-BC, COHN-S
Caroline Koehler, MSN, RN
Leslie Morris, BSN, RN

The worlds of Informatics and Evidence-Based Practice have changed the office visit. Nurses are increasingly challenged to provide nursing care and patient education using the most up-to-date practices. Electronic medical records (EMR) allow sharing of information across nursing and medical disciplines and can incorporate patient participation. The patient may have access to portions of the medical record and be able to communicate with medical personnel via their personal computers or other electronic devices (e-communicate).

E-communication and Telephonic encounters offer opportunity to speed patient assessment, to reduce face-to-face visits, to increase the types of patient education offerings, and may increase patient safety. An effective EMR will allow connection to electronic safety nets such as medication review and chronic disease registries that can decrease the chance of errors. Nursing practice and office work flows may improve based on the use of electronic schedules, and data collection with analysis. The Internet and Intranets offer volumes of professional literature that can assist in connecting the patient to community resources.

In the midst of the Informatics and Evidence-Based Practice world, the nurse remains challenged to integrate the theoretical and clinical knowledge to plan, direct, coordinate, and evaluate the delivery of quality care. Orientation practices for new employees focus on the assessment, screening, and triage of presenting symptoms and risk factors to deliver effective nursing care and client education (Laughlin, 2006). The nursing process is the keystone for assessment, planning, implementation, evaluation, and documentation of the care and education provided. Appropriate consultation with health team members and utilization of organizational processes will flow from the assessment process. Management of the acute, chronic, or episodic presenting problems need to include consideration of the client's primary language, culture, spiritual and emotional concerns, learning style, educational level, age considerations, sexual preference, and utilization of listening techniques to establish a therapeutic nurse-client relationship.

The degree of independence with which a registered nurse provides or delegates nursing care will be dependent upon state regulations and organizational policies in the area in which the nurse practices. A planned orientation and competency assessment maximizes the success of the nurse in daily practice. Effective orientation and professional development lead to providing clients with quality nursing outcomes and staff retention. These have professional and economic ramifications that can impact the individual nurse and the medical practice area, as well as the patient.

This chapter will reflect the professional nursing role in the most common areas of ambulatory nursing practice. Key components of the topics have been defined and examples are provided in chart form so you may select from the menu to create a plan that fits your organization and individual work setting.

1. **Dimension: Primary Care and Adult Health**
   Core Curriculum for Ambulatory Care Nursing, 2nd ed. (Laughlin, 2006, pp. 237-285, 321-382).

   Definition:
   Primary care is the provision of integrated, accessible health care provided by clinicians who develop a sustained partnership with patients in creating a medical home (Institute of Medicine [IOM], 1996, p. 5)

   Introduction:
   Ambulatory health care occurs in a wide variety of settings. Primary care covers the continuum of life, embracing all cultures and socioeconomic groups. The main objective of primary care is prevention and health maintenance.

   Key Action Tips:
   - Health maintenance and prevention are necessary for all age groups.
   - Assessment skills are required of ambulatory nurses.
   - Educate patients.
   - Document in the medical records.
   - Offer multicultural care.
   - Provide customer service.

   Example:
   Marcella and Jose Garcia have two children, Emilio and Anna. Mrs. Garcia arrives at the pediatrician's office with her 8-year-old son, Emilio, for his well child exam. It is the family's first visit to this office. Mrs. Garcia has limited English. Emilio speaks English fluently. In preparing for the physician exam, Emilio has his height, weight, and vital signs taken. His BMI is determined to be 27. A vision screen determines that Emilio has a visual acuity of 20/40. A telephone line with an interpreter service is contacted and an interpreter is used to assist in obtaining demographics, family history, and health history. The nurse discovers that Emilio is behind in his immunizations. Spanish versions of the handout for 8- to 10-year-olds on developmental milestones and personal safety, VIS (Vaccine Information Sheets) forms for delayed immunizations, dietary information, and nutritionist referral are gathered in anticipation of an education session with the RN following the physician visit. Mrs. Garcia is encouraged to bring Anna in for her well check-up and to update her immunizations.

Subtopic	Elements	Competency Statement
Primary Care/Family Practice	➤ Well baby checks ➤ Childhood immunizations schedules ➤ School and sports physical ➤ Male/female adult well physical recommendations (PSA, prostate exam, mammogram, Pap, fecal occult blood, colonoscopy) ➤ Triage and assessment of complaint or condition ➤ Respond quickly to emergent conditions such as acute coronary syndrome, abdominal pain, stroke ➤ Participates in stabilization and prepares patient for transport to acute care ➤ Routinely obtains allergy medication and medical history	Collaborates with other health team members, utilizing organizational, federal, professional group clinical guidelines, protocols, and standards of practice in providing care to patients exhibiting frequent and high-risk conditions encountered in the practice setting.

Subtopic	Elements	Competency Statement
Physical Assessment Skills for Evaluation of Complaint/Condition	➤ Auscultation, observation, palpation, percussion of body cavities and extremities *Equipment:* • EKG/cardiac monitor • IV insertion and therapy • Infusion devices • Laboratory studies • Opthalmoscope/otoscope • Oxygen administration/pulse oximetry • Pain assessment/scale • Pharmacotherapeutics • Point of care testing (blood glucose monitor, rapid step, urine dip stick) • Sharps management • Spirometry • Stethoscope • Vital signs, height, weight, BMI • Department-specific equipment and procedures	Provides assessment techniques utilizing current tools, screening methods, and resources to determine appropriate care for commonly encountered disease states and emergency situations.
Client Education	➤ Printed materials, Web sites, class schedules, anatomy and physiology charts and models, organizational and community resources • Interpreter service for native language • Identify behavior/knowledge goals • Provide return demonstration opportunities for use of equipment • Contract provided for follow-up and subsequent concerns of problems • Identifies significant others present with the client • Validates patient information and demographics • Incorporates the nursing process	Uses active listening skills to determine the knowledge base of the patient and responds with an appropriate language level when providing information and instructions.
Documentation in the Medical Record	➤ Identifies the process and resources used in the provision of care • Consultations • Guidelines, protocols, and standards of care • Printed materials • Physical assessment findings • Diagnostic and screening test results • Pertinent cultural issues • Education needs • Service and referral decisions • Follow-up plans • Client agreement or non-agreement ➤ Maintains confidentiality of the medical record	Provides multiple education resources in varying formats that best suit the client's needs. Documentation meets organizational, professional, and accreditation standards in facilitation communication of the patient condition in the provision and coordination of treatment and services.

Subtopic	Elements	Competency Statement
Customer Service/Cultural Competency	➤ Interpreter service for native language • Provides instructions in written format using native language whenever possible • Assists team members to provide culturally sensitive care • Maintains confidentiality of the encounter	Applies customer service principles in the work setting. Adapts clinic routines to accommodate language and cultural preferences.

Adult Health/Patient Prototypes: Hypertension	➤ Risk factor identification:
	• Family history
	• Risk behaviors
	• Patient demographics
	➤ Physical assessment:
	• Vital signs
	• Height and weight, BMI
	• Reviews of prior B/P reading and trends
	• Heart sound
	• Associated symptoms
	• Lifestyle behaviors
	➤ Prevention measures:
	• Lifestyle modifications
	• Medication therapy with nutritional education
	• Provide for home monitoring of B/P
	• Regularly scheduled physical examinations
	➤ Patient education incorporates:
	• Determination of target B/P lifestyle management
	• Exercise
	• Weight management
	• Avoidance of nicotine use
	• Stress management
	• Medication use and purpose
	• Hypertensive emergencies
	  – Severe headache
	  – Mental status changes
	  – Vision changes
	  – Limb numbness
	  – Generalized weakness
	  – Chest pain, palpitations
	  – Shortness of breath
	  – Dizziness, facial drooping
	• Outcome management:
	• Medication compliance
	• B/P at target or below
		Assesses, screens, and triages to identify hypertension, particularly in the at-risk population.
		
		Advocates for the client by providing primary, secondary and tertiary prevention, education, and community resources as needed.
		
		Develops an ongoing care plan that provides regular monitoring and physical examination with laboratory studies to conserve target organs of heart, brain, eyes, and kidneys.

Subtopic	Elements	Competency Statement
Adult Health/Patient Prototypes: Hypertension (continued)	• Weight control • Increased exercise tolerance • Decreased dietary sodium, fat, and cholesterol intake • Avoidance of nicotine	

Diabetes Mellitus	➤ Risk factor identification:
	  • Obesity
	  • Disease history in a first degree relative
	  • Ethnic background of African American, Native American, Hispanic, Asian
	  • Prior gestational DM
	➤ Secondary prevention interventions:
	  • Blood glucose control
	  • Lipid management
	➤ Tertiary interventions:
	  • Management of complications of eyes, nerves, kidneys, and heart
	➤ Physical assessment:
	  • Blood glucose and lipid monitoring
	  • Foot exam for skin integrity, circulation status, sensitivity, and deformities
	  • Blood pressure
	➤ History assessment:
	  • Physical activity
	  • Diet
	  • Medication compliance
	➤ Education outcomes:
	  • Verbalizes the disease process and the purpose of medication therapy
	  • Performs accurate blood glucose monitoring and maintains retrievable records
	  • Maintains target blood glucose level
	  • Compliant with medication administration
	  • Maintains diet and exercise routines
	  • Describes hypoglycemia and treatment intervention
	  • Recognizes symptoms appropriate for contacting health care provider
	  • Maintains treatment plan
	➤ Intervention outcomes:
	  • Patient participates in own care
	  • Conservation of eyes, nerves, kidneys, and heart
		Describes types of diabetes and associated risk factors.
		
		Assesses, screens, and triages patients with diabetes utilizing basic diabetes knowledge and skill to teach patient competencies.
		
		Advocates for the patient through patient/family education, proper referral services for classes, complex management of disease, and other coexisting chronic conditions.

Subtopic	Elements	Competency Statement

Heart Failure	➤ History taking:
	• Cardiac, diabetes, thyroid, and anemia history
	• Cardiac surgery/invasive procedures
	• Lifestyle
	  – Alcohol and nicotine use
	  – Excessive fluid, sodium, fat intake
	  – Activity level
	  – Stress management
	  – Medication compliance
	  – Medication history
	➤ Physical assessment:
	• Vital signs, heart sounds
	• Venous neck distention
	• Dyspnea, orthopnea, paroxysmal nocturnal dyspnea, cough, rales
	• Weight gain
	• Peripheral edema, change in mental status, dizziness
	• Nausea, anorexia
	➤ Education outcomes:
	• Hypertension control
	• Lipid control
	• Cessation of smoking and alcohol use
	• Improved exercise and stress management
	• Weight control and monitoring weight
	• Limited sodium dietary intake
	• Medication compliance
	• Self-management of dietary, fluid, and exercise routines
	➤ Ongoing care:
	• Annual flu vaccine and senior pneumococcal immunization
	• Regular physical examinations
	• Prompt recognition and seeks treatment of worsening condition
	• Identification and treatment of exacerbating conditions
		Conversant with the anatomy and physiology of heart failure, current therapies and interventions, and the homodynamic goals of therapy.
		
		Advocates for the patient/family with disease state education and referral to patient organizations for psychosocial and disease management issues.

Subtopic	Elements	Competency Statement
Chronic Obstructive Pulmonary Disease	➤ History taking: • Risk behaviors • Demographics • Occupational factors • Morning sputum • Acute chest illness history ➤ Physical assessment: • Chest auscultation • Observation of position of comfort, respiration characteristics, and accompanying accessory muscle use • Chest x-ray • Spirometry with bronchodilators • Arterial blood gas studies ➤ Prevention interventions: • Smoking cessation • Medications/Metered Dose Inhalers (MDI) • Pulmonary rehabilitation • Oxygen therapy ➤ Education outcomes: • Smoking cessation • Compliant with therapies • Manages MDI, oxygen delivery systems independently • Avoids exacerbating activities, exposures • Seeks appropriate medical assistance with worsening condition	Discusses the current definitions for the traditional diagnoses of emphysema, COPD, and chronic bronchitis. Educates the patient/family in lifestyle modifications to slow or reverse the disease process. Assists the patient in understanding medication therapies and monitoring tools that assist with managing the disease processes.
Prevention: Diet, Exercise, and Sleep Pattern	➤ Nutritional status (diet): • Body Mass Index (BMI) • General appearance of face, eyes, oral cavity, skin, hair, nails, posture, muscle tone, reflexes • Abdominal and neck palpation • Diet history ➤ Exercise: • History • Activities of daily living • Exercise routines • Mobility limitation	Promotes general well-being and health through assessment and education for diet, exercise, and sleep pattern.

Subtopic	Elements	Competency Statement
Prevention: (continued) Diet, Exercise, and Sleep Pattern	➤ Sleep: • History • Lifestyle demand/stress • Non-pharmacologic methods to encourage sleep • Education resources provided for diet, exercise, and sleep appropriate to age group ➤ Education outcomes: • Patient is able to set initial personal goals for weight, exercise, and regular sleep pattern	

Substance Abuse	➤ History of current and past use of substances leading to chemical dependency; inability to fulfill major role obligations at work, school, or home; social/ interpersonal problems associated with effects of the substance
	• Alcohol
	  – Drinks per day
	  – Alcohol behavior routines
	• Prescription drug overuse
	• Street drugs
	  – Amphetamines
	  – Cocaine, crack cocaine
	  – Heroin
	  – Marijuana
	  – Others
	  – Method of use
	➤ Assessment
	• Nutritional status
	• Needle scars
	• Rhinorrhea from nasal inhalation
	• Blood alcohol level
	• Toxicology screens
	➤ Education and resources
	• Age and culturally appropriate printed and video materials
	• Options for care
	➤ Educational outcomes
	• Seeks appropriate medical and behavioral health care
		Obtains history to determine current and past substance abuse of patient or primary care giver.
		
		Collaborates with patient, health care provider, and community resources to offer substance abuse care.
		
		Assures health referrals for related cardiac, vascular, respiratory, and other substance abuse-related diseases.

Subtopic	Elements	Competency Statement

Substance Abuse (continued)	➤ Tobacco use
	  • Assessment
	    – Current and past patterns of tobacco use
	    – Smoking cessation history
	    – Number, types, and lengths of prior attempts
	    – Reasons for quitting
	    – Causes of relapse
	    – Readiness to change
	  • Educate patient on the consequences of tobacco use
		Assess patient use of tobacco products. Educate regarding the health risks related to tobacco use and suggest approaches for cessation with possible referral to tobacco cessation programs.

Prevention – Disease	➤ Breast cancer screening
	  • Family history, surgical history
	  • Clinical exam yearly for women over 40, every 3 years for women 20-39
	  • Mammogram yearly starting at age 40 (unless high risk)
	  • Education
	    – Role of exercise and nutrition in the prevention of breast cancer
	    – Self-breast exam techniques
	    – Self-breast exam monthly starting at age 20
	➤ Cervical cancer screening
	  • Family history
	  • Pelvic exam every 1-3 years with Pap test for sexually active women
	  • Education
	    – Sexually transmitted herpes virus (HPV) infections and cervical cancer
	    – Risk reduction behaviors
	    – Immunization options
	➤ Colorectal cancer screening (see women's health and male health sections)
	  • Risk factors
	    – Family/personal history of colorectal cancer of polyps
	    – Personal history of inflammatory bowel disease
	    – Obesity
	    – Poor nutrition
	    – Screening for age 50 and older
	    – Fecal occult blood test (FOBT) for fecal immunochemical test (FIT) yearly or flexible sigmoidoscopy (FSIG) every 5 years
	    – Annual FOBT or FIT and FSIG every 5 years or double contrast barium enema every 5 years or colonoscopy every 10 years
		Obtains age-specific breast, reproductive, and respiratory tract cancer observations and risk history to provide appropriate screening, referral, and education.
		
		Obtains age-specific colorectal cancer risk history to provide consultation and referral for appropriate screening detection and education.

Subtopic	Elements	Competency Statement
Prevention – Disease (continued)	➤ Hearing and vision • History/surgery • Related medical history • Regular examinations for hearing and visual acuity • Ophthalmic glaucoma screening and retinal health • Ultraviolet ray reduction sunglasses for cataract prevention • Noise exposure	Encourages age-specific screening of hearing and vision. Promotes use of adaptive equipment to increase hearing and visual acuity.
	➤ Nicotine use history (see substance abuse section) ➤ Osteoporosis • Assess for risk factors of age diet exercise, history of fracture at age younger than 50, history of hip fracture, diminished height, kyphosis • Bone density • Baseline at age 60 or older	Provides education and referral to patients identified for osteoporosis risk.

	➤ Skin cancer screening
	• Appearance for vascularity, lesions, texture turgor
	• Avoid sum-seeking behavior and tanning salons
	• Wear protective clothing
	• Use sunscreens and UV protective lip balm
	• Use protective measures with children and infants
	• Regular examination of all skin surfaces such as recognition of suspicious lesions including melanoma using "ABCDs"
	• Education: instructs about risk factors, signs and symptoms of skin cancer
	• Appearance of hair – color, texture, and distribution
	➤ Immunizations
	• CDC recommendations – schedules (www.cdc.gov/vaccines)
	  – Infant
	  – Child
	  – Adult
	• Screen for contraindications to immunizations
	• Patient education – Vaccine Information Sheets (VIS)
	• Control and prevent epidemics of vaccine preventable diseases
		Uses well client/family visits as an opportunity to discuss the prevention and early detection of skin cancer. Encourages regular examination of all skin and scalp surfaces and skin cancer screening as a regular part of the patient physical exam.

Subtopic	Elements	Competency Statement

Prevention – Injury	*Risks by age group:*
	➤ Infants
	  • Burns
	  • Falls
	  • Infection
	  • Ingestion/inhalation of foreign objects
	  • SIDS
	  • Suffocation/drowning
	➤ Toddler/preschool
	  • Burns
	  • Falls
	  • Guns/weapons
	  • Lacerations
	  • Ingestion/inhalation of foreign objects
	  • Suffocation/drowning
	➤ School age
	  • Burns
	  • Drowning
	  • Guns/weapons
	  • Fractures
	  • Inhalation/ingestion of foreign objects
	  • Motor vehicle accidents
	➤ Adolescent (see adolescent care)
	  • Drowning
	  • Guns/weapons
	  • Inhalation/ingestion of foreign objects
	  • Motor vehicle accidents
	➤ Adult
	  • ETOH (ethanol), nicotine, drug use
	  • Domestic violence/abuse
	➤ Seniors
	  • Burns
	  • Falls
	  • Medication overdose
	  • Motor vehicle safety
		Collaborates with patient and health team members to promote a safe living environment for all developmental age groups.

Subtopic	Elements	Competency Statement
Prevention – Injury (continued)	➤ Education outcomes include appropriate use of: • Seat restrains for motor vehicles • Child-proofed home including locked cupboards for caustic substances and drugs, gates at stairway, avoidance of wheeled vehicles near stairwells • Fire extinguishers/smoke alarms/CO detector in working order • Electric outlet covers • Access to poison control phone number • Guns/weapons are unloaded, trigger lock is in place and activated • Continuous supervision of young children around water ➤ Education includes information on safety equipment, drug, alcohol, sexuality, sexually transmitted diseases, and birth control	Collaborates with patient and health team members to promote a safe living environment for all developmental age groups.

Prevention – Oral Health	➤ Poor oral health and its effect on the quality of life
	• Risk factors
	  – Low income socioeconomic status
	  – Uninsured or under insured for dental health
	  – Culture of ignoring dental disease
	  – Later children in family with high caries incidence
	  – Demonstrated caries; fillings, plaque, staining
	  – Sleeping with a bottle or breast fed through the night
	• Education
	  – Dental caries is a preventable, communicable disease caused by streptococcus mutans
	• Consequences of poor oral health and lack of treatment
	  – Altered appearance and speech
	  – Poor nutritional status due to pain, poor dentition
	  – Reduced self-esteem, social interaction, education and career advancement
	  – Families with high caries incidence
	  – Seven-fold increase in low birth weight babies of pregnant women with periodontal disease
	  – Increased incidence of cardiovascular disease and stroke
		Identifies high-risk individuals for oral caries and communicates the consequences of poor oral health.

Subtopic	Elements	Competency Statement

Prevention – Oral Health (continued)	➤ Low birth weight infant prevention
	  • Streptococcus mutans bacteria colonize the infant between 6-30 months
	  • Hormonal changes during pregnancy increase acid uric bacteria, thus increasing caries, gingivitis, and periodontal disease in the pregnant woman
	  • Low birth weigh infants are at high risk for cerebral palsy, mental retardation, and blindness
	➤ Dental caries prevention
	  • Oral cavity assessment
	    – Infant oral exam between 6-12 months or eruption of first tooth
	    – Buccal mucosa, gums, teeth, tongue, salivary glands
	  • History bottle use
	    – Oral surgery
	    – Dental care routine
	    – Oral hygiene routine
	    – Oral nicotine use, smoking
	    – Diet assessment of adequate calcium phosphorus, vitamin D
	  • Education outcome
	    – Adequate oral hygiene practice
	     - Stannous fluoride dentifrice/varnishes/sealants
	     - Daily flossing
	    – Diet adequate in calcium, phosphorus, vitamin D
	  • Reduced/eliminated alcohol and nicotine use
	  • Positive response to oral health referral
		Provides education to the pregnant woman on the relationship between periodontal disease and low birth weight infants.
		
		Encourages oral health through assessment, education, and referral to increase general health.

2. Dimension: Pediatrics

Definition:
The branch of medicine that deals with the medical care of infants, children, and adolescents.

Introduction:
Pediatrics covers the continuum of life from birth to 18-years-old. Children are seen in pediatrics for prevention visits and sick visits. Cultural competency and excellent customer service are two important aspects of a pediatric visit.

Key Action Tips:
- Practice health maintenance and prevention.
- Display assessment skills.
- Focus on patient/caregiver education.

Example:
Mrs. Schultz arrives at the pediatrician's office with her 2-year-old daughter, Ruth. Ruth is fussy with audible stridor. Ruth's mom states the child has been having "noisy breathing since late last night." Ruth's vital signs are within normal limits. Her weight and pulse oximetry are taken. The pulse ox reads 92%. The registered nurse takes a complete data collection and does a physical assessment prior to the physician exam.

Subtopic	Elements	Competency Statement
Well Child Visit	➤ Well baby/child checks ➤ School and sports physicals ➤ Utilizes age appropriate information and screening tools: • Patient's age • Caregiver's name and relationship to patient • Reason for visit • Pertinent/additional symptoms • Vital signs • Pulse oximetry, as applicable • Weight and height percentile • Body mass index percentile • Head circumference, as applicable • Assess tobacco use of patient and/or caregiver(s) • Vision screening • Age appropriate diagnostic screening tests (PKU, PPD, spirometry, peak flow) • Review medical-surgical history • Review social history • Review chronic health problems • Review allergies • Review current medications • Last menstrual period, as applicable • Review and update immunization history	Provides anticipatory guidance and screening procedures to promote wellness for enhanced growth and development of the well child.

Subtopic	Elements	Competency Statement

Well Child Visit (continued)	➤ Immunizations
	  • CDC recommendations – schedules (www.cdc.gov/vaccines)
	    – Infant
	    – Child
	    – Adult
	  • Screen for contraindications
	  • Patient education – Vaccine Information Sheets (VIS)
	➤ Control and prevent epidemics of vaccine preventable diseases
	➤ Knowledge of the stages of growth and development
	➤ Abuse/domestic violence assessment
	➤ Provides information/education for appropriate age:
	  • Nutrition and elimination
	  • Sleep and activity needs
	  • Psychosocial requirements
	  • Safety recommendations
	  • Parenting tips
	  • Healthy habit recommendations
		Delivers care appropriate to the child's developmental level with consideration of the caregiver's education and culture.

Equipment and Data Collection for Evaluation of Complaint and/or Condition	➤ Equipment:
	  • Stethoscope
	  • Blood pressure cuff, appropriate size
	  • Sphygmomanometer
	  • Thermometer
	  • Opthalmoscope/otoscope
	  • Pulse oximetry
	  • Peak flow meter
	  • Spirometry
	  • Tape measure
	  • Scale
	  • Vision screening charts
	➤ Data collection:
	  • Name
	  • Age and gender
	  • Name and relationship of adult accompanying child
	  • Vital signs, height, weight, BMI
	  • Head circumference, as applicable
	  • Chief complaint	

Subtopic	Elements	Competency Statement
Equipment and Data Collection for Evaluation of Complaint and/or Condition (continued)	• Signs and symptoms related to chief complaint • Other accompanying symptoms, as applicable • Onset of symptoms • Duration/pattern • Pain assessment/scale • Medical-surgical history • Chronic health problems • Allergies and adverse medication reactions • Current medications • Birth control type and name, as applicable • Last menstrual period, as applicable • Recent travel history, as applicable • Self/home treatment and effects, including OTC or herbal remedies	

Asthma Visit	➤ History focus:
	  • Age
	  • Symptoms
	  • Degree of distress
	  • Mental status
	  • Onset/duration
	  • History of asthma or first episode of wheezing
	  • Related signs and symptoms
	  • Current medications
	  • Peak flows
	  • Home treatment
	  • Possible triggers
	  • Frequency of episodes
	➤ Physical assessment:
	  • Vital signs
	  • Pulse oximetry
	  • Observation and assessment of head, neck, chest, and abdomen
	  • Spirometry and peak flow monitoring
	➤ Child and/or caregiver education
	  • Disease process
	  • Medications and their administration
	  • Home monitoring tools
	  • Home treatment plan
	  • Maintaining an active life
	  • Minimizing trigger exposures
	  • Managing a flare
		Provides evidence-based nursing care to the patient with asthma symptoms. Educates the patient and family about asthma.

Subtopic	Elements	Competency Statement

Croup Visit	➤ History focus:
	  • Age
	  • Symptoms
	  • Onset/duration
	  • Related signs and symptoms
	  • Current medications
	  • Medical history
	  • Home treatment attempted
	  • Fluid intake
	  • Activity level
	➤ Physical assessment:
	  • Vital signs
	  • Mental status
	  • Respiratory status
	  • Lung sounds
	  • Voice quality
	  • Observation and assessment of head, neck, chest, and abdomen
	  • Patient position
	  • Anxiety
		Provides evidence-based care to the pediatric patient with croup symptoms.

ADHD Visit	➤ Describe the behavior disorder in appropriate lay terminology
	➤ Educate the family and the community:
	  • Define the behavior disorder at home, in school, and other settings
	  • Describe the rationale for the screening tools
	➤ Collaborate with the health care team in conducting/arranging screening tests and long-term follow-up care:
	  • Identify the disorder through the use of screening tools from parents and teachers
	  • Monitor medications and associated laboratory tests
	  • Provide behavior management techniques
	  • Provide methods to support academic achievement
	  • Provide follow-up while on medication
		Incorporates community resources to support the child and family efforts in managing behavior.

3. **Dimension: Adolescent Care**

Wong's Nursing Care of Infants and Children, 7th ed. (Hockenberry, 2003, Chapter 1, pp. 5-29, Chapter 19, pp. 802-838, Chapter 20, pp. 839-868, Chapter 21, pp. 869-870).
Principles and Practice of Psychiatric Nursing, 8th ed. (Stuart & Laraia, 2005, Chapter 37).

Definition:
Adolescent care involves the physical assessment, health education, screenings, and interventions for individuals who are in transition between childhood and adulthood. Puberty is the biological change that separates childhood from adolescence.

Introduction:
Adolescence is defined as the ages between 11 and 20 during which time bodies and minds experience the hormonal effects of puberty and develop coping mechanisms in response to those changes. The end of adolescence is a reproductively mature adult who has achieved a mature male or female social role, mature social relations with peers, accepted their physical body, and is preparing for a career and other adult/social responsibilities.

There are several health issues that may affect American adolescents. These include the rapid rise in obesity and hypertension continuing from childhood or beginning in adolescence, eating disorders, and personal safety issues related to abuse, firearms, street drugs, and alcohol.

This age group is particularly sensitive to their physical changes and social acceptance by peers and may be skeptical of adult intervention in their lives.

Key Action Tips:
- Include both physical assessment and social history in the data collection.
- Active listening and empathy are important in developing trust with the adolescent to obtain accurate information.
- Special areas for consideration include obesity/eating disorders, intentional self-injury, unintentional injury, physical activity, sexually transmitted diseases, unintended pregnancy, abuse, school and learning problems, and immunization status.
- Health education includes personal safety actions to prevent injury, such as use of helmets, seat belts, and designated drivers.

Example:
Ella, a 14-year-old, is scheduled for her August school physical. Her mother accompanies her. Ella quietly cooperates with you as she is roomed for her physical. She measures 5'3", weighs 152 pounds, and her BMI is calculated at 27. Ella will enter the 9th grade, which will be her first year in high school. She does not seem excited about high school. What additional physical and social assessments will you make? What screening tests would be appropriate? What education might you provide to Ella and her mother?

Subtopic	Elements	Competency Statement

Well and Sick Visit Screening for Risk Factors of Unhealthy and Unsafe Lifestyle	➤ History taking:
	  • Home/environment
	    – Living arrangements
	    – Family relationships
	    – Presence of abuse or violence in the living situation
	    – Culture/ethnicity
	  • Education/employment
	    – Academic status
	    – Community involvement
	    – Work
		Assists in the data collection of the Health Data Information Set (HEDIS) measures to determine need of intervention by self, family, health care, education, or community to promote adolescent health.

Subtopic	Elements	Competency Statement

Well and Sick Visit Screening for Risk Factors of Unhealthy and Unsafe Lifestyle (continued)	• Eating (Caloric Equilibrium)
	  – Diet
	• Activities
	  – Friendships
	  – Recreation
	  – Peer group
	• Drugs
	  – Alcohol
	  – Prescription
	  – Street
	  – Nicotine use
	• Sexuality
	  – Abuse
	  – Identity
	  – Intimacy
	  – Safe practices
	• Suicide
	  – Depression
	  – Intentional injury
	• Safety
	  – Immunization status
	  – Seat belts
	  – Firearms	

Physical Examination Screening	➤ Physical exam:
	• Affect
	• Physical development and fitness
	• BMI
	• Vital signs
	• Cholesterol level
	➤ Immunizations
	• CDC recommendations – schedules (www.cdc. gov/vaccines)
	  – Infant
	  – Child
	  – Adult
	• Screen for contraindications
	• Patient education – Vaccine Information Sheets (VIS)
	➤ Control and prevent epidemics of vaccine preventable diseases
		Utilizes interview techniques that ensure confidentiality and privacy and promote trust with the adolescent.

Subtopic	Elements	Competency Statement

Acne	➤ History taking:
	  • Level of adolescent's distress
	  • Current/past management including OTC, home, and herbal remedies
	  • Perceived success of treatment
	➤ Education:
	  • Physiology
	  • Therapeutic management instructions
	  • Treatment is long-term
	    – Medication information/instructions
	  • When to contact health care provider
		Evaluates the need for medical referral for acne.
		
		Educate and encourage the patient and family to follow the treatment plan for acne.

Caloric Disequilibrium	➤ Obesity
	➤ Eating Disorders
	  • Anorexia Nervosa (less than 85% expected weight)
	  • Bulimia
		Participates in data collection from the adolescent/family regarding dietary intake and activity levels.
		
		Evaluates the need for behavioral health or specialty clinic referral.

Reproductive System Problems, Male	➤ History taking (see adult male health section) ➤ Education (see adult male health section)	Provides an interview technique that promotes trust and confidentiality in order to collect personal data for reproductive health care/prevention. Coordinates developmentally appropriate education and teaching resources for the adolescent.
Reproductive Problems, Female	➤ History taking (see women's health section) ➤ Education (see women's health section)	Provides an interview technique that promotes trust and confidentiality in order to collect personal data for reproductive health care/prevention. Coordinates the education and teaching resources that are developmentally appropriate for the adolescent.

Female Gynecologic Examination	➤ Indications
	  • Menstrual disorders
	  • Undiagnosed abdominal pain
	  • Sexually active
	  • Request for contraception
	  • Suspected pelvic mass
	  • Requested by patient
	  • Rape
	  • 18 years of age
		Identifies the indications explicit or implicit for the need of a pelvic examination.
		
		Arranges procedure setup that meets the emotional needs of the adolescent female undergoing a gynecologic exam.

Subtopic	Elements	Competency Statement

Female Gynecologic Examination (continued)	➤ Education
	  • Presence of support person
	  • Explanation of procedure
	  • Personal hygiene
	  • Physiology
	  • Sexuality
	  • Findings of the exam
		Coordinates education and teaching resources for the adolescent undergoing a gynecologic exam.

Menstrual Problems	➤ Menstrual irregularities history taking:
	  • Physical development
	  • Weight
	  • Eating habits
	  • Vigorous activities
	➤ Dysmenorrhea history taking:
	  • Menstrual
	  • Sexual
	➤ Physical exam
	  • GI system review
	  • GU system review
	  • Pelvic exam possible
	➤ Education
	  • Physiology
	  • Management of condition
	  • Medication management
	  • Diet
	  • Exercise
	  • Avoidance of nicotine
		Discusses and educates patients on menstrual problems and their treatment.
		
		Provides education and information resources specific to the patient problem(s).

4. **Dimension: Women's Health/Gynecology**
Core Curriculum for Ambulatory Care Nursing, 2nd ed. (Laughlin, 2006, Chapter 20, pp. 267-285).

Definition:
Gynecology is the specialty of caring for patients with disease of the female genital system, as well as the endocrinology and reproductive physiology patient needs.

Introduction:
According to the World health Organization (WHO), "the numbers of ageing women are increasing worldwide. In the developed nations of the world, women live on average six to eight years longer than men. Life expectancy for women now exceeds 80 years in at least 35 countries and is approaching this threshold in several other countries" (WHO, 2000). This is why women's health is vital throughout the lifespan. "The health of girls and women is affected by developmental, physiological, and psychological age" (National Institutes of Health [NIH], 2009) and requires promotion of health, prevention, and quality of life. For example, "every day, 1,600 women and more than 10,000 newborns die from preventable complications during pregnancy and childbirth. Almost 99% of maternal and 90% of neonatal mortalities occur in the developing world" (WHO, 2008).

Women's health, obstetrics, and gynecology is a dynamic specialty that provides resources, education, wellness, and medical care to attain the best possible level of health for all women in all stages of life. It is an identified special area of emphasis that is being validated by "increased investigation into methods to prevent conditions and diseases, or to better treat them, can result in significant improvements in the quality and length of women's lives. Prevention research spans the continuum from the most basic biological studies to examine the basis of both risk and protective factors and behaviors across the lifespan, as well as the interventions to improve them. This includes a focus on communication of wellness and healthy behaviors in health care provider-patient interactions and in public awareness campaigns" (NIH, 2009). In summary, "there is a very significant scope for improving the health of ageing women and thus ensuring that they remain a resource for their families and communities (WHO, 2000).

Key Action Tips:
* Remain non-judgmental of lifestyle choices of patients.
* Educate to assist the patient in making informed care choices.
* Ask questions and listen; the patient may not know what to report.

Example:
ML calls requesting medication to be called to her pharmacy for a vaginal infection. During the interview and assessment on the phone, the nurse finds that ML indeed has a discharge but also has abdominal pain intermittently, low grade fever, and nausea. The patient is seen by appointment that day and is treated for pelvic inflammatory disease. Patient is instructed on the treatment plan and provided with STD prevention information.

Subtopic	Elements	Competency Statement

Normal Prenatal and Postpartum Care	➤ History taking:
	• Inherited diseases screening
	  – Genetic history of client and partner
	  – Ethnic background
	• Family medical histories
	  – Diabetes
	  – Hypertension
	  – Cardiovascular disease
	  – Kidney disease
	  – Nervous system disease
	  – Behavioral health condition
		Obtains the genetic, ethnic, family, and personal history of the pregnant mother and father.

Subtopic	Elements	Competency Statement

Normal Prenatal and Postpartum Care (continued)	• Personal medical history
	   – Last menstrual period
	   – Blood type, blood transfusions
	   – Thyroid function
	   – Respiratory disease
	   – Cardiac disease
	   – Allergies
	   – Medications
	   – Surgeries
	   – Accidents/injuries
	   – Environmental/medication exposures
	   – Pap test results
	   – STD history
	   – Infertility
	   – Nicotine and alcohol use
	   – Street drug use
	   – Infections since last menstrual period
	   – Immunization status for MMR and Varicella
	➤ Abuse/domestic violence assessment:
	• Observed signs/symptoms
	• Encourage verbalization of history
	• Counseling referral
	• Encourage reporting
	➤ Obstetric history:
	• Gravida
	• Para
	• Miscarriages
	• Abortions
	• Ectopics
	• Living children
	• Pregnancy and postpartum history
	➤ Social history:
	• Educational level
	• Employment
	• Culture
	• Family planning
	• Expectations
	• Abuse/domestic violence	

Subtopic	Elements	Competency Statement

Normal Prenatal and Postpartum Care (continued)	➤ Prenatal education:
	• Travel restrictions after 28 weeks
	• Attend child birth classes in last trimester
	• Maintain good hydration
	• Nutrition
	• Nicotine and alcohol avoidance
	• Exercise
	• Importance of regular care
	• Safe medication use and daily use of prenatal vitamins
	• Pregnancy antepartum and postpartum
	• Complications signs, symptoms, and risks
	  – Hypertension
	  – Diabetes (Type I, gestational)
	  – Anemia
	  – Threatened abortion
	  – Miscarriage
	  – Fetal loss
	  – Hyperemesis
	  – Ectopic pregnancy
	  – Avoidance of communicable diseases
	  – Eclampsia
	  – Placental abnormalities
	  – Multiple pregnancy
	  – Size-date discrepancy
	  – Premature, post date pregnancy
	• When to seek health care
	  – Trauma – MVA or fall
	  – Persistent headache
	  – Vaginal discharge, burning
	  – Vaginal bleeding
	  – Shoulder pain
	  – Burning, pain, bleeding with urination
	  – Persistent, severe vomiting
	  – Fever greater than 100.6° F
	  – Visual changes
	  – Persistent heartburn
	  – Swelling face, hands
	  – Change or decrease in fetal movement
	  – Severe abdominal pain with abdomen tender or rigid, passing clots or tissue
	  – S/S of cool, clammy, faint, or dizzy
		Educates the pregnant patient/family about normal pregnancy, common complications, common procedures, and preparation for labor and delivery.

Subtopic	Elements	Competency Statement
Normal Prenatal and Postpartum Care (continued)	➤ Clinical procedures • Ultrasound • Nuchal translucency • Chorionic villus sampling • Amniocentesis • Group beta strep (GBS) • Fetal movement, non-stress test • Amniotic Fluid Index (AFI) • Biophysical Profile • Fetal fibronectin (FFN) ➤ Childbirth preparation education: • Signs and symptoms of labor • Preterm labor • Directions to the hospital • Childbirth education classes • Breastfeeding resources • Selecting a pediatrician • Options for delivery ➤ Education and care outcomes: • Management of complications • Client seeks health care as appropriate with changes in pregnancy or health • Decrease morbidity/mortality of pregnancy and delivery • Community resource use initiated as needed • Prepared for infant care and safety (car seat) • Attends postpartum visit and follows instructions on sexual relations, family planning/birth control	
High Risk Obstetrics	➤ History taking: • Maternal age, parity, fetal growth • Prior obstetric complications • Preexisting medical problems • Domestic violence issues • Depression (Edinburgh scale) ➤ Education interventions: • Nutrition, nicotine and alcohol avoidance, exercise • Concurrent screening for complications • Specialist referral(s), social services referral	Provides prenatal care for the high risk obstetric patient.

Subtopic	Elements	Competency Statement
High Risk Obstetrics (continued)	➤ Care management coordination for specialty groups, home care, information resources • Individualized plan of care • Cultural considerations	
Perimenopause and Menopause	➤ History taking: • Menses • Signs and symptoms • Hot flashes • Mood swings (depression and irritability) • Irregular bleeding • "Night sweats" • Urinary incontinence • Painful intercourse • Sleep disorders • Vaginal dryness, pruritus • Memory/concentration changes • Domestic violence issues • Intergenerational issues ➤ Prevention interventions: • Annual examination including breast exam, mammogram for age greater than 50 years, pelvic exam, and Pap smear • B/P, height, and weight • Hemocult testing/colonoscopy • Hormone level labs, lipid profile • Bone density measurement • Domestic violence signs/symptoms ➤ Education for lifestyle to promote and maintain well-being: • Provide information on significance of test results ➤ Outcome measures: • Symptom reduction and patient satisfaction • Seeks annual routine care • Participates in care decisions and health maintenance activities • Early detection of cancer, osteoporosis, and heart disease • Reduction in the rate of the above diseases	Provides education on perimenopausal and menopausal states to promote a healthy and active life.

Subtopic	Elements	Competency Statement

Sexually Transmitted Infections	➤ History taking:
	  • Number of sexual partners
	  • Partner history of STDs
	  • Personal history of STDs
	  • Safe sex practices
	  • Pap smear results history
	  • Partner violence
	  • Presence of signs and symptoms
	➤ Assessment:
	  • Unusual vaginal discharge
	  • Culture, Pap smear, wet prep
	  • Colposcopy, biopsy
	  • Blood tests
	➤ Education for prevention:
	  • Treatment information
	  • STD types, signs, symptoms, and no symptoms
	  • Sexual practice with barrier protection for self and partner
	  • Annual health checks
	  • Long-term risks of no or delayed treatment
	  • Infertility
	  • Fetal risk
	  • Recurring flare-ups or outbreaks
	  • Death
	➤ Education and treatment outcomes:
	  • Diagnosis and treatment for client
	  • Assist with arrangements for diagnosis and treatment of partner
	  • Uses appropriate materials that are age, gender, sexual preference, and culturally sensitive
	  • Counseling/education of client and partner
	  • Lifestyle changes implemented
	  • Early detection and treatment of future infections
	  • State reporting completed
		Provides care and preventive education for patients with sexually transmitted diseases.

Subtopic	Elements	Competency Statement
Normal Well Woman Exam – Adult Female Assessment	➤ Age, height, weight, vital signs, LMP, gravida, parity, abortions and living births, last Pap smear, last mammogram ➤ Health maintenance-bone density, lipid profile, mammogram, Td or Tdap, influenza, Pneumovax, flex sigmoidoscopy ➤ Family history – all types of cancer, heart disease, diabetes, HTN, obesity, genetic disorders, and mental health ➤ Current and past medical history, current medications/supplements ➤ Birth control method, drug allergies, surgical history ➤ Discuss and educate on issues such as exercise, smoking, ETOH (ethanol) use, illegal drugs, advance directives, STD prevention and counseling, menstrual cycle, contraceptive counseling, S/S of menopause, osteoporosis prevention, hormone replacement therapy, and breast self-exam ➤ Physical exam that includes breast exam, Pap smear, and pelvic exam	Gathers pertinent medical information, educates the patient about health maintenance, and assists and chaperones the doctor during the exam.

5. **Dimension: Male Health Patient Prototypes**
   Core Curriculum for Ambulatory Care Nursing, 2nd ed. (Laughlin, 2006, Chapter 20, pp. 267-285).
   The Guide to Clinical Preventive Services (Agency for Healthcare Research and Quality [AHRQ], 2006, pp. 11, 43, 50).

   Definition:
   Male health care involves the prevention and treatment of genitourinary conditions and associated endocrine disorders.

   Introduction:
   In contrast to much of preventive medicine, a focus of ambulatory care screening for male reproductive conditions is controversial due to the low yield of case findings. Yet bladder cancer is 2-3 times more common in men than women, particularly those who smoke. It usually occurs at age 50 or beyond and currently, there is no adequate screening test. For prostate cancer, the prostate specific antigen (PSA) test has equivocal findings which may lead to increased numbers of biopsies to confirm positive results. While testicular cancer needs immediate attention, regular self-examination does produce enough positive cases to warrant educating men in the technique. The major thrust for patient education on testicular cancer is that when a nodule is noted by the patient or sexual partner, immediate care is sought.

   Reproductive health is of both psychological and physical importance to men. Most functional difficulties begin around age 50 or later. Erectile dysfunction may be caused by various medications. When not medically managed, benign prostatic hyperplasia (BPH) can lead to an acute, painful episode of inability to void due to bladder neck constriction.

   Key Action Tips:
   - Initiate the subject of reproductive health with the patient.
   - Be sensitive to the difficulty of this subject for most men.
   - Use lay terminology and printed diagrams/photos for education on treatment options.
   - Encourage non-smoking and limited alcohol use.

   Example:
   Bud Phillips, 68 years old, has a history of mild-moderate BPH for the past four years. He takes Tamsulosin HCl (Flomax) nightly. This week he has had a head cold and treated it with over the counter antihistamines. He frantically calls your office saying, "I can't pee. It's killing me!" What history will you take? What immediate action is required? What patient education will be needed?

Subtopic	Elements	Competency Statement
Benign Prostatic Hyperplasia	➤ Symptom history taking: • Dysuria • Urine stream adequacy • Nocturia • Frequency • Double voiding • Dribbling • Changes in symptoms over time and effect on lifestyle ➤ Symptom management education: • Medication compliance • Medication side effects • Symptoms requiring follow-up • Avoidance of spicy foods, salt, caffeine, and alcohol • Voiding completely • Avoidance of OTC products and medications that may increase symptoms	Manages the care and education of patients with benign prostatic hypertrophy.

Subtopic	Elements	Competency Statement

Benign Prostatic Hyperplasia (continued)	➤ Outcomes:
	  • Manages symptoms, reports changes, seeks care as symptoms change
	  • Participates in treatment option decisions
	  • Seeks regular examination	

Prostate Cancer	➤ History for risk factors:
	  • Age
	  • Ethnicity
	  • Family history
	  • Diet high in fat
	  • Vasectomy
	➤ Assessment:
	  • PSA greater than 4
	  • Digital rectal exam
	  • Dysuria, bladder outlet obstruction
	  • Bone pain
	  • General health
	  • Biopsy results
	➤ Education:
	  • Diagnostic tests and treatment options
	  • Preparation for diagnostic tests and procedures
	  • Management of side effects from treatments
	  • Continence/incontinence management
	  • Information resources
	  • Support groups
	  • Terminal care resources
	  • "Red flag" symptoms
	➤ Outcomes:
	  • Participation in diagnostic tests and treatment decisions
	  • Seeks appropriate care for worsening symptoms
	  • Patient/family able to manage side effects
	  • Returns for regular follow-up care
		Provides screening and education of the disease process, symptom management, and treatment options for the patient/family with prostate cancer.

Erectile Dysfunction (ED)	➤ History
	  • Sexual functioning
	  • Medications
	➤ Assessment:
	  • Lab studies
	  • Evaluation of penile anatomy and physiology
		Provides screening and education of the dysfunction process, management, and treatment options for patients with erectile dysfunction.

Subtopic	Elements	Competency Statement
Erectile Dysfunction (ED) (continued)	➤ Education: • Explain the cause of the problem • Support patient through the process of providing explicit sexual function information – lay terminology • Focused listening techniques • Provide information resources • Coordinate care resources • Provide treatment options including medication side effects ➤ Outcomes: • Participation in treatment options • Improved sexual functioning • Adheres to follow-up care plans • Strict confidentiality maintained	
Testicular Cancer	➤ Risk factor history: • Age • Ethnicity • Socioeconomic status • Prior cancer of testicle • Cryptorchidism • Infertility • In utero exposure to DES ➤ Assessment: • Physical exam of testicles • Presence of gynecomastia • Tumor marker lab studies • Imaging studies of pelvis, abdomen, and chest to determine metastatic site ➤ Education outcomes: • Participates in treatment plan • Copes with changes in body image following orichectomy • Adheres to follow-up care plans ➤ Prevention education: • Boys with cryptorchidism should have corrective surgery by age 6 • Prompt attention to a lump or painless swelling of the testicle	Provide education of the disease process, the urgency of prompt treatment, treatment options, and follow-up care for the patient/family with testicular cancer.

6. Dimension: Gerontologic Health
Core Curriculum for Ambulatory Care Nursing, 2nd ed. (Laughlin, 2006, Chapter 20, pp. 267-285).
Assessing and Measuring Caring in Nursing and Health Science, 2nd ed. (Watson, 2008, Chapter 5, pp. 64-81).

Definition:
Geriatric nursing care is provided for individuals who are traditionally 65 and over. However, people feel old based on their health and functional ability, rather than chronologic age.

Introduction:
The 25-30+ year span of geriatrics includes persons who are active, highly functioning, and often still employed to those whose mobility and mentation are highly compromised. There is great variability in the age when a person is more limited in their functional and or mental status. Health issues for the elderly include hypertension, reduced cardiac output, heart murmurs, increased residual urine and urinary tract infections, increased urge incontinence, constipation, sensory deficits, and problems maintaining acid-base balance.

In American culture, the aged often express loneliness and feeling uncared for. For many, their independence is quite important and they are concerned about becoming a burden to family and friends. Demonstrate caring for the geriatric client by active listening to determine the client's concerns, offer education in a respectful manner, involve the patient in their plan of care, and provide touch. Frailty, pain, arthritis, and degenerative conditions may limit how quickly the patient may be able to move or respond to verbal interaction. Demonstrate patience when responses are slow.

Key Action Tips:
- Demonstrate caring behaviors.
- Assess for functionality, depression, mentation, and health status.

Example:
Mrs. Cecelia Adams arrives for her senior care nursing appointment with her son, Harold. Harold states that his mother is still living in her apartment. He is concerned that she has lost weight, doesn't play bridge anymore, and talks repeatedly about her silverware being stolen. You take Mrs. Adams' height, weight, and vital signs.

You obtain a medication history by interviewing her son as well as comparing information from the chart. After doing a physical exam you administer the Mini Mental Status Test, the Geriatric Depression Scale, and the Activities of Daily Living Screen. Over a period of a month you assist the son to locate assisted living accommodations for Mrs. Adams with an on-campus Memory Unit, should that be needed in the future.

Subtopic	Elements	Competency Statement

Health and Functional Assessments	➤ Geriatric Depression Scale
	➤ Mini Mental Status Test
	➤ Activities of Daily Living Screen (ADL):
	  • Functional ADL screen
	  • Instrumental ADL screen
	➤ General health/allergies:
	  • Appearance
	  • Hearing and vision
	  • Nutritional status
	  • Medications/polypharmacy assessment
	  • Management of chronic conditions
	  • Nicotine and alcohol use
	  • Pain
		Screens and educates the older adult on health and functional status to promote a safe and active lifestyle.

Subtopic	Elements	Competency Statement

Health and Functional Assessments (continued)	➤ Safety of living situation:
	  • Driving safety
	  • Food preparation
	  • Personal care
	  • Medication compliance
	➤ Support systems:
	  • Family resources
	  • Financial status
	  • Physical/financial abuse assessment
	  • Community, state, federal resources
	➤ Outcomes:
	  • Safe living situation
	  • Socialization opportunities
	  • Management of chronic conditions	

Health Promotion	➤ Patient/caregiver education:
	  • Nutrition for prevention or decrease of osteoporosis
	  • Medication management for acute and chronic conditions
	  • Exercise program
	  • Pain control for osteoarthritis, cancer, other
	  • Financial resources/support
	    – Self-determination
	    – Attorney in fact
	    – Power of attorney designation
	  • Grief and loss support
	  • Spiritual/personal values support
		Provides information on community resources to assist the older adult patient/family in maintaining or increasing health, an active lifestyle, and a safe living environment.
		
		Encourage completion of Durable Power of Attorney for Health Care, Living Will, and DNR forms to minimize conflicting family viewpoints at end of life.

7. Dimension: Oncology Pain Management
Core Curriculum for Ambulatory Care Nursing, 2nd ed. (Laughlin, 2006, Chapter 23, pp. 389-399).

Definition:
Pain is defined by the International Association for the Study of Pain as "an unpleasant sensory and emotional experience associated with actual or potential tissue damage." It has sensory, affective, cognitive, emotional, and cultural components.

Introduction:
Pain is a subjective experience that is both physiologic and emotional. The person's response is influenced by his or her culture and individual expectations of pain. Standardized pain assessment tools help the patient communicate his or her pain experience and individualize approaches to pain relief. Care providers must be able to recognize physical symptoms of pain when a patient cannot communicate them. Chronic pain affects vital signs, suppresses immunity, and decreases mobility. A major issue in providing pain relief is that many drugs have multiple, unpleasant side effects. Recent research has endeavored to provide complementary therapies in addition to traditional medications. Health care providers must trust the patient assessment of their pain and provide relief appropriate to the patient assessment.

Key Action Tips:
- Ask about pain.
- Observe for non-verbal cues for pain.
- Educate the patient and family on pain and pain relief strategies.
- Believe what patients say about their pain.
- Use a multidisciplinary approach to develop individualized pain relief strategies.
- Reassess pain once interventions are implemented.

Example:
Mrs. Delores Gonzales, age 75, had a left foot amputation last year, secondary to her long history of diabetes mellitus. She continues to experience phantom limb pain for which she has made this appointment. Mrs. Gonzales comes to your clinic with her daughter who is pushing her in a wheel chair. What information, evaluation, and consultation will you do to create a pain relief strategy for Mrs. Gonzales?

Subtopic	Elements	Competency Statement

Pain Assessment	➤ Pain history:
	  • Location
	  • Frequency
	  • Quality
	    – Nocioceptive (tissue damage)
	    – Neuropathic (nervous system damage)
	  • Pattern of pain (constant/intermittent)
	  • Aggravating/alleviating factors
	  • Rating scale
	  • Pharmacologic interventions and results/side effects
	➤ Physical assessment with level of function
	➤ Psychosocial assessment
	➤ Pain classification
	➤ Patient/caregiver education on pain management interventions and side effects
		Screens and educates the oncology patient/family on managing plan.

Subtopic	Elements	Competency Statement
Pain Prevention	➤ Patient/family education to identify causes and interventions that provide relief ➤ Regular medication administration 24/7 ➤ Provide additional medication for breakthrough pain ➤ Distraction with humor, music, mild exercise ➤ Complementary therapies (relaxation, guided imagery, hypnosis)	

Pain Intervention	➤ Distraction
	➤ Premedication for procedures
	➤ Presence of support person
	➤ Noninvasive cutaneous stimulation with heat and cold:
	  • Site location for heat/cold
	  • Prevention of skin damage
	➤ Invasive medication administration:
	  • Subcutaneous administration
	  • IV administration
	  • Intraspinal administration
	    – Patient positioning
	    – Site observation
	    – Monitoring vital signs and neurologic status
	  • Surgical neuroablation
	➤ Provide patient/caregiver education:
	  • Assessment
	  • Interventions
	  • Medication with narcotics and other controlled substances
	  • Medication interactions
	➤ Written instructions for interventions
		Uses the source of pain to determine age-appropriate interventions to manage pain.
		
		Uses professional guidelines for the administration of medications.
		
		Educates the patient/family in effectively managing pain.

Pain Management Outcomes	➤ Patient outcomes:
	  • Recognition of pain and causal factors at the onset
	  • Recognition of warning signs to seek health care
	  • Utilization of preventive and relief measures
	  • Utilization of pain journal to assist in monitoring and modifying interventions
	➤ Professional outcomes:
	  • Prioritization of pain management
	  • Utilization of protocols, guidelines, standards of care
	  • Demonstrate proficiency in assessment and management
		Identifies community resources for services that will support the patient/family in maintaining the treatment plan for pain management.

8. **Dimension: Neurology Patient**
Core Curriculum for Ambulatory Care Nursing, 2nd ed. (Laughlin, 2006, Chapter 21, pp. 312-314).

Definition:
The most common acute neurologic conditions encountered in ambulatory care include headache, back pain, and cerebral vascular accident.

Introduction/Key Action Tips:
- Be alert to red flags for emergent care for all three conditions.
- All three conditions can result in chronic disability.

Example:
A female caller contacts the physician office and speaks to the nurse. She reports, "My husband can't get out of bed. When I ask him what's wrong, he just mumbles, and now he has wet the bed. This has never happened before." What are your next actions? What will you tell the wife?

Subtopic	Elements	Competency Statement
Headache • Tension • Migraine • Cluster • Rebound	➤ History: • Prior history • Age of onset • Frequency • Duration • Location, onset, quality, intensity • Associated symptoms (nausea/vomiting, visual changes) • Trigger • Treatment tried and results ➤ "Red flags" for emergent care: • Confusion, memory loss, neurologic symptoms • Visual problems • Unresponsive to treatment • Stiff neck and illness • "Worst headache ever" • First severe headache ➤ Assessment: • Vital signs • Neurological evaluation ➤ Education outcomes: • Can describe types of headaches • Able to identify and avoid triggering substances, events, environments • Able to discuss medication and non-medication interventions (stress reduction, biofeedback, massage)	Assesses and triages patients with headache symptoms. Recognizes and arranges for emergent care of "red flag" symptoms of a headache. Educates the patient/family on ways to reduce the incidence of headaches.

Subtopic	Elements	Competency Statement
Headache (continued) • Tension • Migraine • Cluster • Rebound	➤ Intervention outcomes: • Able to manage lifestyle to avoid or greatly reduce incidence of headaches • Compliant with preventive medication administration and acute incidence medications	
Back pain	➤ History taking: • Incident activity • Location • Onset • Quality • Alleviating factors/treatment tried • Aggravating factors • Medical and medication history ➤ Physical assessment: • Neurological symptoms ➤ Education and prevention outcomes: • Implements rest, local treatment therapies, exercise as guided by health care team • Seeks appropriate health care with increased symptoms or lack of progress • Return to prior level of activity and work	Identifies symptoms of acute back pain resulting from spinal conditions.

Stroke/Cerebral Vascular Accident	➤ Identifies emergent symptoms:
	• Numbness, weakness of limb(s)
	• Loss of function of any body part
	• Change in mental status
	• Visual disturbance
	• Difficulty walking due to imbalance or dizziness
	• Severe headache of unknown cause
	➤ Lifestyle assessment and education for prevention:
	• Adherence to anticoagulation therapy
	• Nicotine and alcohol use cessation
	• Diet modifications for low fat, low cholesterol intake
	• Weight modification
	• Exercise
	• Stress management
	• Management of coexisting conditions
	   – Hypertension
	   – Cardiac disease, other
	• Able to seek health care for emergent symptoms or rehabilitation complications
		Provides appropriate emergent care for patients with acute stroke.
		
		Assists the patient/family in making lifestyle changes for prevention of future stroke episodes.

Subtopic	Elements	Competency Statement

Stroke/Cerebral Vascular Accident (continued)	➤ Coordinates with community services:
	  • Physical therapy, occupational therapy, speech therapy
	  • Transportation
	  • Psychosocial issues
	➤ Prevention outcome measures:
	  • Progressive improvement in ADL
	  • Successful use of adaptive techniques and devices
	  • Prevention of complications
	➤ Arranges supportive care and nutrition for the terminal patient in the home environment
		Collaborates with the health care team and community services to continue long-term patient follow-up after a stroke.

9. **Dimension: Ambulatory Surgery**
Core Curriculum for Ambulatory Care Nursing (Robinson, 2001, Chapter 19, p. 331).

Definition:
Ambulatory surgery is also known as outpatient surgery or same-day surgery. An Ambulatory Surgery Center (ASC) is a health care facility that provides minor surgery, pain management, diagnostic, and screening endoscopy in an outpatient setting.

Introduction:
There are a broad scope of surgeries performed in ASCs – knee, shoulder, eye, spine, pain management, and endoscopy services. ASCs appeared as an option in healthcare in the 1980s and continue to expand today. There are more than 22 million surgeries a year performed in ASCs across the country. Complications are rare; however, ASCs are required to have a plan for transferring patients to a full-service hospital if the need arises. ASCs are licensed by the state, certified by Medicare, and accredited by a major health care accrediting organization. The main accreditors of ASCs are:
- American Association for Accreditation of Ambulatory Surgical Facilities (AAAASF) – www.aaaasf.org
- Accreditation Association for Ambulatory Health Care (AAAHC) – www.aaahc.org
- The Joint Commission – www.jointcommission.org
Nursing usually has the primary responsibility for maintaining compliance with the standards to acquire and maintain accreditation.

Key Action Tips:
- Schedule patients with a health status of ASA 1, 2, or 3.
- Pre-operative instructions are provided in the physician's office or by telephone.
- Laboratory and testing clearances are completed prior to the procedure.
- Check chronic illness control to prepare for procedures.
- Financial arrangements should be made in advance.

9. **Dimension: Ambulatory Surgery (continued)**

Example:
Mary Jane needs a screening colonoscopy. The nurse in the physician's office provides instruction regarding the pre-procedure preparation that is needed and schedules the procedure. The ASC nurse reviews the patient's history and finds Mary Jane has diabetes. The patient's recent blood glucose and hemoglobin A1C are reviewed and are found to be in a safe range. The nurse consults with the physician and contacts the patient regarding diabetes medication management for the day of the procedure. The ASCs business office contacts Mary Jane to discuss insurance coverage and fees she will be responsible for and to arrange for a payment plan if needed.

On the day of the procedure, Mary Jane is prepared for the procedure in the pre-op area of the ASC. A finger stick glucose is assessed and documented. Anesthesia is made aware of the patient's diabetes and its control. Following the procedure, the nurse in post-op recovery checks the patient's glucose. It is 68; the patient complains of feeling shaky and four ounces of juice is given. The glucose level is monitored until discharge.

Patient and family members are given post-procedure instructions by the nurse with time allowed for a question and answer period. Emergency phone numbers are provided, precautions are given regarding when and how to call if having difficulty, and emphasis is placed on the need for Mary Jane to eat a meal and return to normal medication routines as soon as possible.

Subtopic	Elements	Competency Statement

Care Coordination for Adult and Child	➤ Pre-operative instructions:
	• Information resources on the procedure
	• Informed consent
	• Insurance forms, pre-authorization
	• Lab/imaging or other studies
	• Anesthesia interview
	• Self/home preparation prior to procedure
	  – Diet/NPO
	  – Bowel prep
	  – Skin prep
	  – Medication management
	• Location of surgery facility
	• What to wear (jewelry and personal items are discouraged)
	• Need for driver for safe discharge
	• Notification of facility if ill day of surgery
	• Financial responsibilities
	  – Insurance reimbursements
	  – Medicare standards
	  – Payment at time of service or payment plan
	➤ Recovery information:
	• What to expect in the immediate post-op period
	• Family visitation
	• Discharge requirements
		Provides pre-operative instruction to the patient and family.
		
		Provide post-operative instruction to patient and family or other designee.

Subtopic	Elements	Competency Statement
Care Coordination for Adult and Child (continued)	➤ Discharge/home care instructions: • Diet • Self-care • Care of the operative site • Medications • Pain management and pain medications, • Personal hygiene (bathing, showering) • Signs of infection, bleeding • When to seek care prior to scheduled follow-up • Activity level and limitations • Adjunctive therapies ➤ Return to normal activities (driving, housework, job) ➤ Referral to patient organizations for psychosocial support ➤ Arrange follow up care (office, home, or other facility) ➤ Referral to community, state, federal agencies for financial support	
Knowledge and Skill Set	➤ IV access and medication administration ➤ Cardiac and oxygen monitoring ➤ Availability of age appropriate equipment ➤ Sterile field preparation and maintenance ➤ Knowledge of surgical instrumentation, cleaning, sterilization ➤ Support to the surgical team: • Instrumentation and procedure supplies management • Ability to function in an emergency • Equipment and supplies are available and maintained • Roles and responsibilities are designated through collaboration with surgical team members • Personally provides care during an emergency ➤ Monitors patient in recovery: • Utilizes professionally recognized guidelines for care and discharge • Alert to untoward anesthesia effects • Vital signs, cardiac, and oxygen monitored • Surgical site assessed • Pain managed • Discharge per Aldrete (or other) score • Provide post-op follow-up calls to assess status and answer questions	Assures support procedures and operative room set ups are appropriate for each given operation.

Subtopic	Elements	Competency Statement

Education	➤ Assesses readiness to learn, provides motivating information if seems fearful or not interested
	➤ Determines what the patient/family already knows or understands
	➤ Utilizes guidelines, protocols, standards of practice in providing information and modifies according to individual need (age, language)
	➤ Provides for pre-operative facility tour if possible, showing expected equipment to be encountered pre- and post-operatively
	➤ Provides written instruction/information that is in native language when possible
	➤ Utilizes interpreter services as needed
	➤ Has patient repeat information to determine level of understanding
	➤ Uses focused listening skills to determine additional concerns or learning needs
	➤ Provides for return demonstrations when appropriate
	➤ Assesses family need for support services
	➤ Education outcomes:
	  • Cooperative and calm patient/family
	  • Reduction in complications
	  • Adherence to postoperative instructions
	  • Seeks health care appropriately post-operatively
	  • Returns for follow-up care as directed
	  • Utilizes adjunctive therapies as directed
		Provides the patient/family with information about the surgical procedure that is appropriate to the age level and education level.
		
		Modifies care throughout the operative stages to meet the cultural requirements of the patient/family.

Conscious Sedation	➤ Screening for appropriateness for patient according to age, general health, procedure scheduled
	➤ Emergency equipment is available:
	  • Pediatric and adult resuscitation equipment and medications
	    – Oxygen source and back-up
	    – Bag valve mask
	    – Suction equipment
	    – Battery-powered back-up illumination
	    – Vital sign, oximetry, and cardiac monitors
	    – Cardiac defibrillator
	    – Mechanism to summon help
	  • Regular maintenance of equipment
	  • Regular practice with equipment
	  • Roles and responsibilities for emergency resuscitation are designated
		Assesses and triages patients scheduled for conscious sedation.
		
		Provides emergency resuscitation for problems associated with conscious sedation.

Subtopic	Elements	Competency Statement

Conscious Sedation (continued)	➤ Familiar with drug actions, side effects, monitoring and reversal procedures
	➤ Patient education (see education section)
	➤ Discharge per Modified PAR (post-anesthesia recovery score) or other
	➤ Outcomes:
	  • Satisfied patient
	  • Ability to return to pre-procedure level of functioning or better
	  • Compliant with home care instructions
	  • Attends follow-up visits
	➤ Documentation:
	  • Reflects standards used in providing care
	  • Education
	  • Patient response to services and interventions
	  • Discharge criteria
	  • Patient follow-up plans
		Uses standard proceedings to deliver care, monitor condition, and discharge the patient having conscious sedation.

10. Dimension: Nurse-Managed Clinics: Patient Prototypes
Core Curriculum for Ambulatory Care Nursing, 2nd ed. (Laughlin, 2006, Chapter 3, p. 40).

Definition:
Nurse-managed clinics can be geographic or department specific. It is a practice where all nursing care is directly controlled by the nurses.

Introduction:
Nurse-managed clinics have increased the availability of outpatient health care to members of society. Depending upon the state nurse practice act and the individual nurse's practice, the clinic may be independent or part of a health care practice or organization where there is physician and other health services collaboration. The nurse is aware of third party reimbursable expenses in providing cost-effective care.

Key Action Tips:
- Collegial work environment with physicians and nurses managing patient populations.
- Advanced practice nurses must comply with the state's rules and regulations where they work independently.
- The nurse will support the medical model through written protocols.

Subtopic	Elements	Competency Statement

Wound Care Clinic	➤ History assessment:
	• Wound history/causative factors
	• Risk factors
	   – Diabetes
	   – Peripheral neuropathy
	   – Autoimmune disease
	   – Cardiac disease
	   – Vascular insufficiency
	   – Other chronic conditions
	     - Obesity
	     - Poor nutritional status
	     - Sedentary lifestyle
	     - Immobility
	     - Decreased mentation
	     - Incontinence
	     - Increasing age
	     - Long-term steroid therapy
	     - Infectious agent
	     - Recent surgery or trauma
	• Medical-surgical history
	• Medications and allergies
		Functions within the state nurse practice act to coordinate the care of chronic, acute, and surgical wounds.

Subtopic	Elements	Competency Statement

Wound Care Clinic (continued)	➤ Physical assessment:
	• Wound size, depth, condition, location, drainage
	• Evaluation of surrounding tissue
	• Vital signs, height, and weight
	• Mobility and balance; need for assistive devices
	• Cardiovascular status
	• Respiratory status
	• Wound culture and CBC with differential
	➤ Interventions:
	• Topical therapy
	  – Remove necrotic tissue
	  – Eliminate infection
	  – Eliminate air space
	• Absorb excess exudate
	  – Insulate the wound bed
	  – Protect from trauma/contamination
	  – Maintain moist environment
	• Dressings
	  – Transparent film
	  – Polyurethane foam
	  – Gauze
	  – Hydrogel
	  – Hydrocolloids
	• Pharmacological management
	  – Antibiotics
	  – Steroids
	  – Pain medications
	  – Diuretics
	• Lifestyle management
	  – Diet (high protein) to promote wound healing and compatible with other health conditions
	  – DM blood sugar control
	  – Peripheral edema management
	  – Address sleep, rest, positioning
	• Living and support services evaluated with facilitation of addition support systems as needed
		Provides education on community resources or refers the patient/family for in-home care as needed.
		
		Educates client/family on the wound condition, management, and desired outcome of wound care.
		
		Encourages family participation in providing direct care when possible and to assist with lifestyle changes necessary to promote wound healing.

Subtopic	Elements	Competency Statement

Wound Care Clinic (continued)	➤ Education outcomes:
	  • Knowledge of causative factors
	  • Maintains follow-up visits
	  • Compliant with medications
	  • Improves nutritional status
	  • Avoidance of nicotine and alcohol
	  • Complications avoided or minimized
	  • Wound improves and closes	

Anticoagulation Clinic	➤ Risk factor assessment:
	  • Coagulation disorder
	  • Recurrent thrombosis
	  • Cardiac disorders
	  • Allergies and current medications
	➤ Screening assessment:
	  • Medical-surgical history
	  • Physical exam
	  • Vital signs, height, weight, BMI
	  • Nutrition and lifestyle
	  • Cognitive ability
	  • Mobility (fall history)
	  • Dexterity
	  • Available support system
	➤ Pharmacotherapeutics:
	  • Heparin
	  • Low molecular weight heparin
	  • Warfarin
	  • Assessments for nutritional supplements, OTC medications, and prescribed medications with anticoagulant effect
	➤ Education outcomes:
	  • Therapeutic INR range maintained
	  • Prevention and management of bleeding
	  • Has printed information on medication, desired effect, side effects, prevention of bleeding, importance of follow-up appointments, and lab studies
		Functions within the state nurse practice act to collaborate with a physician in assessing, screening, and managing patients receiving anticoagulation medication.
		
		Utilizes guideline or protocol to evaluate and monitor patients receiving anticoagulation therapy.
		
		Provides education to maximize patient understanding and compliance with medication and laboratory monitoring to produce a safe and effective anticoagulant state that is personally satisfying to the client.
		
		Educates patients to maintain an effective anticoagulant state.

Subtopic	Elements	Competency Statement
Anticoagulation Clinic (continued)	➤ Collaborates with patient/family/resource services to provide needed support: • Meals • Transportation • Finances • Interpreter needs • Aware of cultural impact on therapy compliance and requested lifestyle modifications	

Incontinence/Continence Clinic	➤ Risk factor history:
	• Medical-surgical and obstetric history
	  – Chronic lung disease
	  – Neurologic disorders
	  – Chronic bowel disease
	• Age
	• Diet high in spices, acids, caffeine
	• Fluid intake minimal
	• Nicotine and alcohol use
	• Constipated bowel pattern requiring routine intervention
	• Impaired mobility
	• Impaired cognition
	• Allergies and medications, OTC drugs, and herbal preparations
	➤ Assessment:
	• Symptoms of urinary incontinence (UI)
	  – Frequency
	  – Urgency
	  – Leakage
	  – Nocturia
	  – Retention
	  – Overflow
	• Examination of genitals and integument
	• 24-hour I and O log
	• Suprapubic fullness
	• Palpation of hard stool in the abdomen, bowel sounds
		Assesses patients to determine the type and causes of incontinence.

Subtopic	Elements	Competency Statement
Incontinence/Continence Clinic (continued)	➤ Education/outcomes: • Has printed information that describes the problem and lifestyle interventions to support bladder health and continence • Lifestyle changes are initiated/maintained to support bladder health and continence • Uses a toileting schedule as appropriate • Bladder training • Use of assistive devices • Use of containment devices • Intact perineal integument • Improved continence or containment ➤ Collaboration: • Patient/family/resource services • Meals • Transportation • Finances • Interpreter needs • Aware of cultural impact on behavioral compliance and requested lifestyle modifications	Educates the patient/family to prevent, control, or reduce the degree of urinary incontinence. Identifies community resources to support the patient/family in managing urinary incontinence.

References

Agency for Healthcare Research and Quality (AHRQ). (2006). *The guide to clinical preventative services, 2006.* Rockville, MD: Author.

Hockenberry, M.J. (Ed.) (2003). *Wong's nursing care of infants and children* (7th ed.). St. Louis, Mosby.

Institute of Medicine (IOM). (1996). *Primary care: America's health in a new era.* Washington, D.C.: National Academy Press.

Laughlin, C.B. (Ed.). (2006). *Core curriculum for ambulatory care nursing* (2nd ed.). Pitman, NJ: American Academy of Ambulatory Care Nursing.

National Institutes of Health (NIH). (2009). *FY 2009 NIH research priorities for women's health.* Retrieved from http://www.nih.gov

Robinson, J. (Ed.). (2001). *Core curriculum for ambulatory care nursing.* Philadelphia: W.B. Saunders.

Stuart, G.W., & Laraia, M.T. (2005). *Principles and practice of psychiatric nursing* (8th ed.). St. Louis, MO: Mosby.

Watson, J. (Ed.). (2008). *Assessing and measuring caring in nursing and health science* (2nd ed.). New York: Springer Publishing Company.

World Health Organization (WHO). (2000). *Fact sheet # 252 – Women, ageing, and health.* Retrieved from http://www.who.int

World Health Organization (WHO). (2008). *10 facts about women's health.* Retrieved from http://www.who.int

Additional Readings

American Academy of Pediatrics and the American College of Obstetricians and Gynecologists. (2002). *Guidelines for perinatal care* (5th ed.). Illinois: Author.

American College of Obstetricians and Gynecologists. (2007). *Guidelines for women's health care: A resource manual* (3rd ed.). Washington, D.C.: Author.

Burke, M.M., & Walsh, M.B. (1997). *Gerontologic nursing: Holistic care of the older adult* (2nd ed.). St. Louis: The C.V. Mosby Co.

Chase, H.P. (1995). *Understanding insulin-dependent diabetes* (8th ed.). Denver: Barbara Davis Center for Childhood Diabetes, Dept. of Pediatrics, University of Colorado Health Sciences Center.

Di Mura, C. (2000). Patient education: Enhancing the potential of the teacher and the learner. In N. Burden (Ed.), *Ambulatory surgical nursing* (2nd ed., pp. 363-380). Philadelphia: W.B. Saunders.

Kaiser Permanente. (2007). *Telehealth nursing documentation guideline (revision 2007).*

Kaiser Permanente. (2009). *Nursing guidelines.* Colorado: Author.

Schmitt, B.D. (1991). *Your child's health* (rev. ed.). New York: Bantam Books.

Schmitt, B.D. (1999). *Pediatric telephone advice* (2nd ed.). Philadelphia: Lippincott-Raven.

Wallach, M., & Grimes, D.A. (Eds.). (2000). *Modern oral contraception, updates from the contraception report.* Totowa, NJ: Emron.

Chapter 4

Professional Nurse Role

Linda Brixey, RN
Ann Jessie, MSN, BSN, RN
Wanda Mayo, BSN, RN, CPN
CDR Terrie C. McSween, NC, USN

The role of the professional nurse in the ambulatory care arena is unique in its care approach and setting. Therefore, when orienting a nurse to the ambulatory care setting, it is important to stress the distinctive qualities of the role the ambulatory nurse performs. The professional nurse brings competencies to the work setting such as collaboration, communication skills, advocacy, critical thinking, needs assessment, and program evaluation. An organization that sets the expectation for the nurse to use these skills in his or her ambulatory practice incorporates aspects of each into the orientation program.

Through collaboration, the professional nurse brings the right people together to meet the client's needs and promote continuity of care. Members of the health care team include, but are not limited to, the social worker, various therapists, dietician, pharmacist, physician, and family members and significant others working together to optimize the care plan for the patient.

Through communication, the professional nurse functions in a pivotal role, bringing members of the healthcare team together to ensure the issues related to the patient's plan of care are explored and addressed, and finally executed with the patient, family, and/or significant other. The plan of care can be modified to meet the patient's changing conditions and needs. Patient education in various media is used as a communication tool to improve adherence to prescribed treatment plans.

As an advocate, the professional nurse seeks to represent the needs or wishes of the patient, family members, or significant others to other members of the health care team and assure that the patient's voice is heard.

Critical thinking is the epitome of daily practice. The professional nurse uses the hallmarks of critical thinking by using observation, experience, evidence-based practice, and judgment to prioritize, collect data, problem-solve, assess, evaluate, then reassess to communicate findings in a manner that builds and supports the patient's goal or journey to wellness.

Through continual needs assessment, the professional nurse anchors the patient's plan of care to real needs or concerns of the patient, thus assuring treatment of the whole patient, not just a disease or symptom.

Continual program evaluation of an orientation program for the professional nurse assures the orientation is valid to the practice setting. A "one size fits all" concept of orientation doesn't assure that the needs of the employee or organization are met. A comprehensive orientation should be provided in both a didactic and hands-on learning opportunity, tailored to the unique requirements of the nurse's role within the ambulatory setting, assuring a mutual understanding of professional expectations that are dynamic and ongoing. Professional growth and development using a self-needs assessment format addresses the professional learning needs that will identify opportunities for remediation or enrichment leading to greater professional satisfaction and improved outcomes for patients.

In this chapter, the professional nurse's role is reflected through the dimensions of Competency of the Professional Nurse: clinical process improvement, ethics, leadership, inquiry, research, evidence-based practice, workplace regulatory compliance, staff development, and provider self-care. Key components of each of these topics have been defined and examples of these components are provided. This information is provided here in chart form so you may select from the menu to create a plan that fits your organization and individual work setting.

1. **Dimension: Competency of the Professional Nurse**
"Ambulatory care nurses employ practices that in nature are: restorative... supportive... (and) promotive" (AAACN, 2010, p. 12). Professional ambulatory care nurses employ current nursing knowledge, incorporate evidence-based nursing practices and apply the critical thinking, interpersonal and technical skills necessary to complete their assigned job responsibilities.

Definition:
Professional competence is the "degree to which the individual can use the knowledge, skill, and judgment associated with the profession to perform effectively in domains defined by a scope of professional practice" (Kane, 1992).

Introduction:
Competence for the professional nurse ensures the delivery of safe, effective, and relevant care in a variety of settings. It is the development and the implementation of professional standards, code of ethics, and comprehensive certification programs that denote the commitment to the profession of nursing that ensures continuity and development (Labunski, 2000). Competency is a dynamic process based on the integration of evidenced-based nursing practice, knowledge, and skill that include monitoring and evaluating of performance as a mechanism for feedback on a regular basis.

Key Action Tips:
- Competency testing should be relevant to the professional nurse's position and work setting and assist in the orientation and assignments in unfamiliar work settings.
- Job descriptions should incorporate the expected competencies and objective measures.
- Professional development should not be limited to competency skill test.
- Self-evaluation, assessment tools, and study material must be a part of each educational intervention.

Example:
Professional regulation is demonstrated by:
- Professional credentials
- An unencumbered license
- Performance testing:
  - Checklist of skill inventories
  - Peer evaluations
  - Chart audits
- Objective testing:
  - Standardized examination
  - Certification exams
- Continuing education
- Adherence to Standards for Clinical Practice
- Advanced practice certifications or academic degree(s)
- Evidence-based practice determines what competencies are needed

Subtopic	Elements	Competency Statement

Competency by Integrating Knowledge, Skill, and Ability	➤ Participates in identifying competencies necessary to deliver care
	➤ Evaluates and monitors on a regular basis staffs' competency, incorporating a variety of methods to support performance improvement initiatives
	  • Critical thinking
	  • Collaboration
	  • Communication
	  • Advocacy
	  • Needs assessment
	  • Evaluation
	➤ Practice reflects expertise in the three competency dimensions:
	  • Professional role
	  • Responsibility
	  • Expertise
	➤ Critical thinking: collects and analyzes information in order to arrive at logical, defendable conclusion
	➤ Technical: performs tasks safely
	➤ Interpersonal: influences patient/families and/or health care team members through verbal and nonverbal skills and behavior
		Utilizes the nursing process in performance of assigned duties.

Credentialing and Validation	➤ Verification of credentials
	  • Verification of educational background
	  • Criminal background check
	  • Valid nursing license
	➤ Job description
	  • List of minimum credentials for position
	  • List of essential duties
	  • Core expectations of employee defined
	➤ Assessment of skills competency
	  • Validation of core skills needed for quality care
	  • Chart audit for compliance
	  • Competence across continuum of the health care team and practice setting/specialty
	  • Safe medication administration
	  • Demonstrates safe, effective, and efficient use of equipment needed for patient care
		Maintains required qualifications to perform position duties.

Subtopic	Elements	Competency Statement

Credentialing and Validation (continued)	➤ Patient education
	  • Disease and symptom management instruction
	  • Medication-specific instruction
	  • Medication reconciliation
	  • Equipment use for self-treatment instruction
	➤ Documentation
	  • Complete and timely documentation of signs and symptoms, other pertinent information
	  • Charting meets Joint Commission, NCQA, AAAHC or other regulatory or required standards
	  • Personnel file reflects attendance of required educational programs and updates to meet regulatory requirements and remain competent
	➤ Critical thinking skills
	  • Practices legally and within scope of practice
	  • Risk/problem recognition, management, and prioritization	

2. **Dimension: Clinical Process Improvement**

AAACN Standard 7: Performance Improvement
The performance improvement process is coordinated and integrated with that of the organization and includes the continuous data collection, evaluation, and improvement of the safety, quality and appropriateness of ambulatory care nursing (Laughlin, 2006, pp. 169-172).

Definition:
Performance improvement (PI) is the systematic analysis of the structure, process, and outcomes within systems for the purpose of improving the delivery of care (Joint Commission on Accreditation of Healthcare Organizations [JCAHO], 2005).

Introduction:
Performance improvement is one of the most critical endpoints in a quality model. Without the PI process, nursing cannot adequately meet the demanding needs of the aggressively growing patient population in ambulatory care. The nursing process involves the review of objective and subjective information, assessment of the information received, identification and implementation of a plan to meet the identified need, followed by reassessment to ensure that the plan adequately met the needs that were addressed. The Performance Improvement process applies the same principles as the nursing process, just utilizing a different format.

Key Action Tips:
- Define the problem – (Set Aims).
- Determine that the change is an improvement – (Establishing Measures).
- Identify specific changes that will result in improvement – (Selecting Changes).
- Plan, Do, Study, Act – (Testing Change).
- Pilot the new change – (Implementing Change).
- Share the wealth – (Spreading Change).

Example:
- ID the problem: No standards, no policy.
- Form a steering committee to oversee project and provide the continuous analysis component.
- Create a plan, identify roles and needs of staff, implement steps needed to develop policy, educate staff and check competency, then evaluate if it was successful with or without a pilot group.
- Assess outcomes of the pilot group and, if successful, prepare for implementation across the continuum.
- If not successful, review and implement new steps to address the problem and re-pilot.

Subtopic	Elements	Competency Statement
Performance Improvement (PI) Process	➤ Incorporates PI into practice ➤ Utilizes Plan, Do, Study, Act (PDSA) Model ➤ Systematically utilizes PI methodology to analyze the structure, processes of the care setting, and outcomes within systems to improve delivery of care ➤ Be knowledgeable of the annual performance improvement indicators and supportive report cards ➤ Integrates competencies and multiple, interrelated system and interpersonal factors into cohesive quality improvement action plans ➤ Collaborates with other healthcare disciplines to achieve quality improvement	Demonstrates usage of tools for effective performance improvement within nursing practice by identifying the problem, creating a plan, collecting data, developing and implementing improvements, setting controls, and analyzing ensuring sustainability.

3. **Dimension: Ethics**

AAACN Standard 12: Ethics
"Ambulatory care registered nurses apply the principles of professional codes of ethics that ensure individual rights in all areas of practice" (AAACN, 2010, p. 32).

Definition:
"Ethics is a process defined by accepted and/or acceptable behaviors that promote high standards of practice, providing a benchmark for members of a profession to use for self-evaluation, establish a framework for professional behavior and responsibilities, provides a vehicle for occupational identity and marks of occupational maturity. Ethics is used as an instrument for persuasion both of members of (a) profession and the public. They enhance the sense of community among members, of belonging to a group with common values and a common mission" (Kultgen, 1988).

Introduction:
Nurses have a strong ethical responsibility. The Code of Ethics created by the American Nurses Association (ANA) provides a framework that is explicit for the framework of primary goals, values, and obligations to the profession of nursing. Traditionally, health care ethics have relied on the principles of respect autonomy, beneficence, non-malfeasance, and justice. The code of ethics assesses the principles and responsibilities derived from it that relies on humanist, feminist, and social ethics as well as cultivation of virtues (ANA, 2005, p. 3).

Ethical behavior recognizes the dignity, diversity, and worth of individuals and families; respects individual cultural, spiritual, and psychosocial differences; and applies philosophical and ethical concepts that promote access to care, equality and continuity of care (AAACN, 2005, p. 6).

Key Action Tips:
- Professional ambulatory care nurses function as patient advocates to ensure that quality care is provided.
- The nurse demonstrates advocacy for patient rights and privacy.
- The patient can speak up and voice his or her opinion without recrimination regarding care and services.
- Nurses should promote healthy self-care activities for their patient populations.

Example:
The professional ambulatory care nurse demonstrates ethical behavior by:
- Providing information about advanced directives
- Utilizing connections to community resources
- Adhering to mandates of Patient Self-Determination Act (1991)
- Providing an interpreter
- Respecting and ensuring cultural, spiritual, intellectual, psychosocial, and age-specific issues are reflected in the care of the patient, family, and/or community
- Obtaining informed consent
- Adhering to regulatory, ethical, and professional standards in business and care delivery

Subtopic	Elements	Competency Statement
Differentiates Between Ethical and Legal Issues	➤ Adherence to the standard of care as it relates to participating in the identification and resolution of ethical concerns, utilizing professional codes of ethics within institutional parameters ➤ The Health Insurance Portability and Accountability Act (HIPAA) of 1996 delineates the patient's rights and responsibilities related to confidentiality of information, personal privacy and self-determination (HIPAA definition, HHS Office of Civil Rights) ➤ Differentiates assessment or care delivery and treatment based on client needs; advocates for appropriate care, including working through an appeals process with insurance carriers when needed ➤ Provide a staff mix appropriate to the intensity level of patients as supported by evidence or research-based staffing pattern designed for ambulatory care settings	Comprehends and incorporates ethical behavior into practice.
Laws That Govern Practice	➤ Nurse Practice Act ➤ American Nurses Association (ANA) Code of Ethics for Nurses ➤ ANA Ethics in Nursing: position statement and guidelines ➤ AAACN value statement/ethic codes	Functions within his or her scope of practice as defined by the State Board of Nursing.
Ethical Principles	➤ Communicate work to staff and patients ➤ Provides a voice for patients and educates patients on their rights: Patient's Bill of Rights ➤ Autonomy: self-determination, the freedom to choose one's own course of action, Advanced Directives, or Patient's Proxy ➤ Beneficence: doing good ➤ Non-malfeasance: acting in a way that avoids, harms (either intentional harm or harm as an unintended outcome) ➤ Confidentiality: to protect the patient's and family's right to privacy, guarding information that the nurse or institution holds regarding the patient (HIPAA) ➤ Justice: fair, equitable distribution of resources ➤ Veracity: truth telling ➤ Fidelity: faithfulness	Incorporates legal and ethical principles into nursing practice.

Subtopic	Elements	Competency Statement
Ethical Decision-Making	➤ Gathers relevant information and facts ➤ Identify stakeholders ➤ Determines abilities of stakeholders to make a decision ➤ Desired outcomes ➤ Action development ➤ Evaluation and reassessment of the effect of the action taken ➤ Understands how own values influence decision-making ➤ Avoids interference of personal values on patient's decision-making	Makes decisions based on ethical principles.

4. **Dimension: Leadership**
AAACN Standard 16: Leadership
"Ambulatory care registered nurses demonstrate leadership behaviors in practice settings, across the profession, and in the community" (AAACN, 2010, p. 38).

Definition:
Leading through traits, behaviors, motivations, and choices to effectively influence others (Berman, Snyder, Kozier, & Erb, 2008, p. 1549).

Introduction:
Nurse leaders influence colleagues and direct reports using a variety of leadership styles to accomplish goals. It is not enough to 'be in charge'; a leader influences the team to work toward a goal using their nursing knowledge, expertise, and inspiration and does not dictate. New clinical staff and new graduate nurses need to experience good leadership to feel valued, grow in their professionalism, and avoid dissatisfaction.

Key Action Tips:
• Continually demonstrate leadership and management behaviors that strengthen nursing practice, enhance organizational performance, improve individual and community health outcomes, advance the nursing profession, and recognize and reward leadership behaviors in others.
• Leadership can come from any level of the organization. Nurses given opportunity to lead a committee or small work group can be mentored into development of strong leadership skills (Habel, 2009).

Example:
A new staff member has prior experience in emergency response. She has worked with her preceptor to orient to the unit. The nurse manager recognizes an opportunity to match the new nurse's skills to a familiar role and invites the new nurse to join the emergency response team. The new nurse is still being oriented. It can be a difficult transition moving from the inpatient to outpatient setting. The new staff member may feel unappreciated and not a part of the team because the work drivers and flow are so different. By building on the strengths of the nurse, the team benefits from her expertise and the new staff member is given the opportunity to interface and network with others on the team.

Subtopic	Elements	Competency Statement

Nursing Leadership	➤ Plan and evaluate interventions/programs
	  • Maintain quality care services
	  • Enhance practice
	➤ Act as change agent
	  • Implementation of change
	  • Evaluate change/programs
	  • Uses national guidelines (e.g., National Guideline Clearing House) to innovate practice
	  • Needs assessment
	  • AAACN standard of practice
	➤ Management strategies
	  • Available organizational Policies & Procedures
	  • Reporting structure
	  • Team rapport
	  • Shared governance
	  • Staffing model development that includes patient acuity, facility design, and equipment availability
		Demonstrates leadership skills that support staff and promote quality patient care.

Leadership Skills	➤ Congruence of vision and agenda for leaders and followers ➤ Planning and actions to achieve goals ➤ Staff development ➤ Enhanced practice ➤ Maintenance of quality care services ➤ Evaluation of interventions and programs	Interprets situations to others and engages them to work collaboratively and collectively.

5. Dimension: Inquiry, Research, and Evidence-Based Practice
AAACN Standard 13: Research

"Ambulatory care registered nurses integrate relevant research findings into practice" (AAACN, 2010, p. 33).

Professional ambulatory care nurses value inquiry and actively expand their nursing knowledge by: participating in educational activities, incorporating evidence-based practices, promoting quality of care and performance improvement initiatives, and evaluating, utilizing, and disseminating the findings of relevant nursing, clinical, and health care systems research.

Definition:
Evidence-based practice is the process by which nurses make clinical decisions based on the best available research evidence. Nurses identify an issue, search the literature, evaluate the research evidence, implement best practices, and evaluate the intervention and outcomes.

Introduction:
Pursuing and integrating increased knowledge and current research-based evidence is a professional responsibility, serving to refine the body of ambulatory care nursing knowledge, advance professional nursing practice, optimize patient outcomes, and enhance organizational and system effectiveness.

Key Action Tips:
- Participate in continuous, diverse educational activities related to nursing, allied healthcare, and organizational effectiveness.
- Implement into practice the most cost-effective evidence available for clinical practice and organizational decision-making.

Example:
- Clinical practice guidelines are statements that have been systematically developed to assist nurses in care delivery processes and assist patients and caregivers in making decisions appropriate to specific diseases or health conditions.
- Evidence-based practice supports establishing a framework for performance improvement processes and development.

Subtopic	Elements	Competency Statement
Research Findings Used to Guide Clinical and Ambulatory Care Practice	➤ Knowledge acquisition • Needs assessment • Risk management data • Process improvement data • Internal/external benchmarking • Financial data • Identification of clinical problem • New research or other standards and guidelines ➤ Participation in and conducting clinical and healthcare system research	Participates in research studies and utilizes research findings to improve care.

Subtopic	Elements	Competency Statement

Research Findings Used to Guide Clinical and Ambulatory Care Practice (continued)	➤ Resources
	  • Agency for Healthcare Research and Quality (AHRQ)
	  • National Guideline Clearinghouse (NGC)
	  • Cochrane Database of Systematic Reviews
	  • National organizations (e.g., NIH)
	  • AAACN standards of practice
	  • Institutional Review Board (IRB)
	  • Libraries and Web sites
	➤ Development of evidence-based practice
	  • Develop question
	  • Assemble relevant research and related literature
	  • Design and implement nursing interventions
	  • Monitor and analyze structure and process
	  • Assess use and evaluate outcome data	

Knowledge of Evidence-Based Practice	➤ Conscientiously utilizes current best practice evidence in professional practice ➤ Educates clinicians to best practice ➤ Applies protocols to health promotion for well populations as well as treatment interventions for the chronically or terminally ill ➤ Provides a framework for evaluating the delivery care ➤ Guides resource allocations ➤ Reduces risk of liability	Incorporates evidence-based practice into professional role.

6. **Dimension: Workplace Regulatory Compliance**
    AAACN Standard 14: Environment

    "Ambulatory care registered nurses actively engage in organizational initiatives that create and maintain an internal environment that is safe, hazard-free, ergonomically correct, confidential, and comfortable for patients, visitors, and staff" (AAACN, 2010, p. 35).

    Definition:
    Regulatory requirements are rules and guidelines that are generated by federal and state legislative acts, by requirements of official agencies representing the public as advocates and purchasers of health care services, and standards developed through professional organizations (Laughlin, 2006).

    Introduction:
    Regulatory requirements support and promote continuous quality improvement, prevent errors, and promote patient satisfaction. Professional ambulatory care nurses are responsible for regulatory compliance in the health care settings where they practice.

    Key Action Tips:
    Professional ambulatory care nurses:
    - "Integrate written policies and procedures that relate to confidentiality, infection control, fire, safety, security, harassment, equipment management, hazardous waste handling, and emergency situations into the practice setting" (AAACN, 2010, p. 35).
    - "Actively participate in orientation and ongoing education programs that are current and relative to creating and maintaining a safe, hazard-free, confidential, ergonomically correct, and comfortable work setting" (AAACN, 2010, p. 35).

    Example:
    - Occupational Safety and Health Administration (OSHA) sets workplace safety and health standards and inspects workplaces for compliance.
    - Americans with Disabilities Act (ADA) protects persons with a disability from discrimination in employment, state and local public accommodations, commercial facilities, transportation, and telecommunication.
    - The Joint Commission is a not-for-profit organization that evaluates and accredits health care programs based on standards that improve the quality and safety of the care provided by (Laughlin, 2006).

Subtopic	Elements	Competency Statement
Compliance to Regulatory Requirements	➤ Adheres to accepted practice and regulatory standards that apply to the practice of ambulatory care • National Patient Safety Goals and Standards • CMS – Centers for Medicaid and Medicare • National Committee for Quality Assurance (NCQA)	Complies with governing body rules and regulations in providing quality care.

Subtopic	Elements	Competency Statement

Compliance to Regulatory Requirements (continued)	• Health Plan Employer Data and Information Set (HEDIS)
	  − Local − fire and building codes
	  − State − scope of practice standards
	  − National − OSHA, HIPAA, Americans with Disabilities Act (ADA), The Joint Commission, CDC, National Committee for Quality Assurance (NCQA), and Accreditation Association for Ambulatory Health Care (AAAHC)
	  − Minimize potential liability
	• Data collection, knowledge of requirements, and role	

Risk Management	➤ Know the 5 steps of risk management:
	  • Identify risks
	  • Options for managing risk
	  • Select risk management options
	  • Implementing options
	  • Monitoring effectiveness
	➤ Assess and reduce risks for patients, staff, and visitors
	➤ Follow organization's policies and procedures
	  • Worker's compensation
	  • Sexual harassment
	  • Advance directives
	  • Patient confidentiality − HIPAA
	  • Patient complaint process
	  • Patient rights and advocacy
	  • Occurrence reporting
	  • Organization's compliance plan
	➤ Appropriate delegation
	➤ Practicing within scope of practice and in compliance with licensing state's Nurse Practice Act
		Implements risk-management strategies in performance role.

7. **Dimension: Staff Development**
AAACN Standard 8: Education
"Ambulatory care registered nurses attain knowledge and competency that reflects current ambulatory care nursing practice" (AAACN, 2010, p. 28).
- Participating in educational activities.
- Incorporating evidence-based practices.
- Promoting quality of care and performance improvement initiatives.
- Evaluating, utilizing, and disseminating the findings of relevant nursing, clinical and health care systems research.

Definition:
Staff development is a specialty of nursing practice defined by standards, based on research, and critical to quality patient and organizational outcomes (National Nursing Staff Development Organization [NNSDO], n.d.).

Introduction:
The art and science of nursing staff development is to promote the image and professional status of nursing, as well as encourage and support nursing research and the application of research findings into practice for the enhancement of healthcare outcomes.

Orientation and continuing education programs, competency assessment, and process improvement activities are key components of staff development. The new staff or graduate nurse is oriented to the new position by being precepted and competencies assessed related to technical skills, critical thinking, and interpersonal communication necessary to perform the expected job duties.

Key Action Tips:
- Transition into professional practice is characterized by the acquisition of the skills, knowledge, and behaviors needed to successfully nurse.
- Lack of preceptoring or comprehensive orientation can cause new nurses to feel disconnected. This leads to turnover or leaving the profession.
- Mentoring of nurses new to ambulatory care practice is essential for successful transitioning.

Example:
A structured orientation program integrating classroom and clinical time eases the transition. Nurses new to ambulatory care have many skills that translate into their new position. The new skills required in ambulatory care practice can cause the nurse to doubt her competency. An orientation that provides a didactic forum which allows the nurse to know what is expected and clinical time with a preceptor can smooth the transition and allow for a successful transition.

Subtopic	Elements	Competency Statement
Personal/Professional Development	➤ Identify barriers and develop strategies to overcome them ➤ Seek professional-based development ➤ Participate in continuing nursing education: local, state, and national levels ➤ Membership and participation in professional nursing organizations	Engages in activities to maintain and enhance professional competence.

Subtopic	Elements	Competency Statement

Staff Development	➤ Facilitates continual learning activities to meet the constantly changing demands of the ambulatory care setting and varied needs of the professional nurse
	➤ Apply adult learning theory in staff development activities
	➤ Utilizes creative methods for learning
	➤ Embraces the 3 competency domains
	  • Psychomotor
	  • Critical thinking
	  • Interpersonal
	➤ Provide professional development
	  • Role development
	  • Effective means for influencing policies and shaping trends
	  • Standards for clinical competency
	➤ Provide access to continuing nursing education: local, state, and national CNE resources and expectations
		Equates quality of care to continual learning, development, and competency of care providers.
		
		Promote ongoing learning activities to develop and maintain staff competencies.

8. Dimension: Provider Self-Care

Definition:
Provider self-care is the examining and nurturing of oneself to maintain a homeostasis within that creates harmony within the mind, body, and spirit.

Introduction:
Caregivers often work under demanding and stressful conditions, where life hangs in the balance. To meet the challenges of the systems within which nurses work, it is imperative that the nurse is self-aware, recognizing those things that may need to be fixed, nurtured, or jettisoned to remove stress. Identifying stress releasers or self-care activities for the mind, body, and spirit can help increase the nurse's potential and performance throughout the work day. The skill of communication is sharpened, enabling the nurse to be a better collaborator, and advocate for those that are placed in his or her care. Critical thinking thrives in an environment that is well-balanced. The contributions that the nurse can make to the patients, work environment, and community are therefore enhanced.

Key Action Tips:
- By caring for yourself, you are caring for your patients, your organization, and your family.
- Identify self-care activities for the mind, body, and spirit.

Example: Staff Conflict
- Write in a journal what occurred with the staff member identifying emotions and concerns.
- Take a walk at break time for 10 minutes.
- Discuss with a friend or confidant.
- Re-evaluate and create a plan for how to address conflict.

Subtopic	Elements	Competency Statement
Benefits of Self-Care	➤ Improved health ➤ Improved job satisfaction ➤ Improved job performance ➤ Ability to balance personal and work life	Works to maintain, promote, and improve personal wellness.
Life Balance and Self-Care	➤ Commitment: dedication to oneself, one's work, and one's family that provides the individual with a sense of belonging and life purpose ➤ Control: empowerment or self-control that helps one overcome elements in the environment so one does not feel victimized ➤ Challenge: ability to see change and problems as opportunities for growth rather that threats to one's existence	

Conclusion

The professional nurse role in ambulatory care incorporates the AAACN *Scope and Standards of Practice for Professional Ambulatory Care Nursing* (2010) with the skills of collaboration, communication, advocacy, critical thinking, needs assessments, and program evaluation to deliver safe and caring nursing care. To ensure the nurse has the skills and knowledge to perform all these skills, orientation and training are essential.

References

American Academy of Ambulatory Care Nursing (AAACN). (2005). *A guide to ambulatory care nursing orientation and competency assessment.* Pitman, NJ: Author.

American Academy of Ambulatory Care Nursing (AAACN). (2010). *Scope and standards of practice for professional ambulatory care nursing* (8th ed.) Pitman, NJ: Author.

American Nurses Association (ANA). (2005). *Code of ethics for nurses.* Retrieved from http://www.nursingworld.org/MainMenuCategories/EthicsStandards/CodeofEthicsforNurses.aspx

Berman, A.J., Snyder, S., Kozier, B.J., & Erb, G. (2008). *Kozier & Erb's fundamentals of nursing: Concepts, process, and practice* (8th ed.). Upper Saddle River, NJ: Prentice Hall Health.

Habel, M. (2009, January 26). Spreading your wings: RNs have what it takes to be effective leaders. *Nurse Week, South Central,* pp. 26-30.

Joint Commission on Accreditation of Healthcare Organizations, The (JCAHO). (2005). *Comprehensive accreditation manual.* Oakbrook Terrace, IL: Joint Commission Resources.

Kane, M. (1992). The assessment of professional competence. *Evaluation and the Health Professions, 15*(2), 163-182.

Kultgen, J. (1988). *Ethics and professionalism.* Philadelphia: University of Pennsylvania Press.

Labunski, A.J. (2000, Dec.). Continuing professional competence [Electronic version]. *Chart.* Retrieved from http://www.findarticles.com

Laughlin, C.B. (Ed.). (2006). *Core curriculum for ambulatory care nursing* (2nd ed.). Pitman, NJ: American Academy of Ambulatory Care Nursing.

National Nursing Staff Development Organization (NNSDO). (n.d.). *NNSDO web page.* Retrieved from https://www.nnsdo.org/

Additional Readings

Hackbarth, D., Haas, S., Kavanaugh, J., & Vlasses, F. (1995). Dimensions of the staff nurse role in ambulatory care: Part 11 – Comparison of role dimensions in four ambulatory care settings. *Nursing Economic$, 13*(3), 152-160.

Institute for Healthcare Improvement. (n.d.). *How to improve: Improvement methods.* Retrieved from http://www.ihi.org/IHI/Topics/Improvement/ImprovementMethods/HowToImprove/

Koerner, B. (1987). Clarifying the role of nursing in ambulatory care. *Journal of Ambulatory Care Management, 10*(3), 1-7.

Titler, M., Kleiber, C., Steelman, V., Rakel, B.A., Budreau, G., Everett, L.Q., et al. (2001). The Iowa Model of evidence-based practice to promote quality care. *Critical Care Nursing Clinics of North America, 13*(4), 497-509.

Chapter 5

Telehealth Nursing Practice

Charlene Williams, BSN, RN, BC, MBA
Sue Olsson, BSN, RN-BC

Telehealth nursing as a component of clinical nursing practice is defined as, "nursing practice using the nursing process to provide care for individual patients or a defined population over a telecommunication device" (AAACN, 2007). It includes any telehealth encounter (via the telephone, Internet, email, or through other electronic technologies) that results in assessment and management of acute and episodic health care concerns, health maintenance and promotion, disease prevention and management, patient education and counseling, patient advocacy, case management, and coordination of care for patients throughout the health care system (AAACN, 2007).

The nurse engaged in telehealth, as in all areas of nursing practice, uses the nursing process to establish a therapeutic nurse-client relationship, which encompasses client assessment, planning, and implementation. This is accomplished through the provision of information, referral, education, support, evaluation, and documentation (Canadian Nurses Association [CNA], 2000). Telehealth nursing practice is primarily associated with the ambulatory care setting and as part of an integrated health care system it enhances existing health care services "to improve access, appropriate use, and efficiency of health care services" (CNA, 2000). In addition as an extension of the clinical setting, it has its own set of assessment, communication, documentation, and evaluation techniques (AAACN, 2007).

Considered to be a subspecialty by the American Academy of Ambulatory Care Nursing (AAACN) and the American Nurses Association (ANA), telehealth nursing practice has its own set of standards that were initially developed by AAACN in 1997 and revised again in 2001, 2004, and 2007. Nurses involved in telehealth nursing practice are required to have specialized nursing knowledge and skills, including at least 3-5 years of demonstrated competence in all aspects of nursing care and independent decision-making. Nursing competencies include strong clinical knowledge and assessment skills, demonstrated by the ability to accommodate age-specific groups, excellent communication skills, and interaction with multiple diverse customers. In addition, technological skills, such as how to operate a keyboard in a Windows application, as well as adapting to other telecommunication equipment relevant to the practice, are required for expertise and performance in telehealth nursing practice.

In this chapter, the professional nurse's role is reflected through the dimensions of telehealth nursing practice, including Technical Skills, Professional Knowledge, Interpersonal Skills, Documentation, Personal and Professional Development, Resource Management, and Issues. Key components of each of these topics have been defined, and examples of these components are provided. This information is in chart form so you may select from the menu to create a plan that fits your organization and individual work settings.

1. **Dimension: Telehealth Nursing Practice/Technical Skills**
Telehealth Nursing Practice Standard III: Competency
Core Curriculum for Ambulatory Care Nursing, 2nd ed. (Laughlin, 2006).
Telehealth Nursing Practice Essentials (Espensen, 2009, Chapter 1, p. 5).

Definition:
"Telehealth nursing is the delivery, management, and coordination of care and services provided via telecommunications technology within the domain of nursing"
(Espensen, 2009, p. 5).

Introduction:
Within most telehealth care settings, time with the patient is very limited compared with other health care settings. The nurse is expected to establish an instant trusting relationship with the patient using communication, charisma, and appropriate interpersonal skills (Espensen, 2009, p. 9).

Key Action Tips:
Use technology to more efficiently utilize the nursing process:
- Develop competency to efficiently use email, word processing programs, databases, and spread sheets.

Example:
- Selection of relevant and appropriate Web-based patient education materials to assist in self-care.
- Nursing involvement in the development and/or adaptations of new technologies to improve patient care, or to deliver care more efficiently.
- Uses computerized flow charts and documentation tools.

Subtopic	Elements	Competency Statement
Telecommunication Technologies	➤ Telephones ➤ Computers ➤ Email ➤ Internet ➤ Facsimile and copiers ➤ Patient portals	Efficiently uses technology to perform role.
Software Programs	➤ Disease management programs ➤ Health information systems ➤ Physician referral modules ➤ Physician to physician consult modules	Understands, selects, and uses relevant software programs appropriately.
Care Management & Analysis	➤ Protocols ➤ Algorithms ➤ Guidelines	Uses selected program decision support tools to address caller/patient needs in order to identify actual and potential health risks. Writes or contributes to the development of protocols and guidelines using current standards of evidence-based practice.

2. **Dimension: Telehealth Nursing Practice/Professional Knowledge**

"Through use of a strong knowledge base, critical thinking skills and articulation of formal nursing guidelines, the nurse is able to advise the patient of the appropriate plan of care, instruct the patient in self-care as appropriate and offer other measures necessary to ensure the best outcome" (Espensen, 2009, p. 24).

Definition:

"To function effectively in all nursing arenas, the nurse must possess the ability to utilize critical thinking and knowledge-based judgment in every patient encounter" (Espensen, 2009, p. 184). The nurse uses electronic devices to communicate with the patient and to receive information from the patient and to monitor his or her condition. Technology is a tool used by the professional nurse rather than a substitute for sound nursing judgment.

Introduction:

Within most telehealth care settings, time with the patient is very limited compared with other health care settings. The nurse is expected to establish an instant trusting relationship with the patient using communication, charisma, and appropriate interpersonal skills (Espensen, 2009, p. 9).

Key Action Tips:
- Assess: interview, collect data, assess, prioritize.
- Plan: determine and use most appropriate decision support tool(s), reference other resources as appropriate, and collaborate.
- Implement: problem-solve, apply intervention and/or activate disposition, educate the patient and/or family, provide support, coordinate resource, and facilitate appropriate follow-up care.
- Evaluate: document, communicate, and perform follow-up analysis (Espensen, 2009, p. 11).

Example:

The nurse controls the call. The patient may call with a self-determined diagnosis. While the nurse needs to respect the patient's opinion, he or she must keep an open mind to other options. Use critical thinking to determine how and why the patient came to the diagnosis. What are the symptoms or other related symptoms? Listen for verbal and non-verbal clues. Consider all the possibilities. A mother calls wanting to determine if it is OK to give prune juice to her 3-month-old for constipation. The nurse asks questions to determine if constipation is the problem. When was the last BM? Was the BM normal? What is the status of the child (fretful, content)? What does the baby eat (bottle or breast)? Any changes in appetite? The nurse is able to determine that the baby is being breast-fed, last BM was 3 days ago but soft and normal, the baby is eating well, and is very happy and contented. The child is not constipated. Using evidence-based guidelines, the nurse determines this is normal bowel patterns for a breast-fed baby (Williams, 2008). Had the nurse just accepted the mother's diagnosis, the wrong care would have been provided.

Subtopic	Elements	Competency Statement
Call Processing	➤ Assessment ➤ Planning ➤ Implementation ➤ Evaluation ➤ Documentation	Manages clinical calls using the nursing process.

Subtopic	Elements	Competency Statement
Assessment	➤ Systematically assesses and addresses patient's needs with decision support tools: • Elicits reason for the call (e.g., chief complaint) and quickly identifies emergent signs and symptoms • Obtains history of symptoms, associated symptoms, allergies, and medical history • Determines priorities • Uses active listening skills • Collects and interprets data • Validates patient/caller information • Keeps encounter client-focused and time-limited	Demonstrates critical thinking skills in assessing covert as well as overt parameters relevant to the needs of the caller.
Planning	➤ Utilizes problem-solving skills ➤ Develops a collaborative plan of care with patient/caller ➤ Employs coaching as needed	
Implementation	➤ Implements plan of care ➤ Gives support and guidance ➤ Provides care advice to caller/patient specific to their needs: • Consultation • Triage • Referrals • Coordination of care	
Evaluation	➤ Elicits caller feedback and evaluates understanding of recommended advice ➤ Follow-up and evaluation ➤ Surveillance	
Age-Specific Competencies	➤ Applies knowledge of growth and development in customer interactions: • Toddler – 1-3 years • Preschool – Child 3-6 years • School Age – Child 6-12 years • Adolescence – 12-18 years • Early Adulthood – 18-44 years • Middle Adulthood – 45-64 years • Late Adulthood – Over 65 years	Provides care consistent with the functional requirements of the person's developmental age.

3. **Dimension: Telehealth Nursing Practice/Interpersonal Skills**

Definition:
"The professional nurse must efficiently establish a caring, trusting relationship with the caller and elicit information related to the reason for the call and current symptoms. After assessing and making a triage decision, the nurse must be able to put closure on the call by summarizing symptoms discussed and repeating health advice given" (Espensen, 2009, p. 9).

Introduction:
"Within the telehealth nursing practice, clear and understandable communication becomes especially challenging because the nurse and the caller cannot observe non-verbal behaviors as a means to confirm the understanding or misunderstanding of the message" (Espensen, 2009).

Key Action Tips:
- Be aware of cultural, ethnic, gender, and racial differences and their potential to impact patient outcomes.
- The professional nurse works to safeguard patient trust by maintaining confidentiality.

Example:
- Follow-up calls after triage or admission to the emergency room.
- Use of interpreter services for patients as necessary.
- Provision of culturally competent care through developing awareness of own knowledge, biases, and skills; the nurse seeks opportunities to broaden awareness of different cultures.

Subtopic	Elements	Competency Statement
Customer Service	➤ Establishes a therapeutic relationship: • Interacts with caller/patient in a warm and friendly manner (courteously greets caller, uses a pleasant tone of voice, displays a calm professional demeanor, etc.) • Establishes level of caller/patient's knowledge • Provides means of overcoming identified barriers to learning • Clarifies and interprets the caller/patient's description of symptoms • Demonstrates ability to adapt to different personalities and emotions • Maintains confidentiality of interaction	Manages clinical calls using the nursing process.

Subtopic	Elements	Competency Statement
Trust-Relationship	➤ Fosters trust: • Identifies self by name and title to the caller • Calls patient by name and/or identifies patient's relationship to the caller • Determines relationship of patient to provider (patient/non-patient) • Immediately takes the necessary actions to meet the caller's requests or needs • Uses simple, direct language for better caller/patient understanding • Listens to understand what the caller/patient has to say • Offers caller the opportunity to express any concerns/problems prior to ending the call	Establishes a trust-relationship to elicit accurate patient/caller information.
Communication Skills	➤ Conducts assessment and focuses on listening, probing, questioning, and analyzing to identify what the caller/patient wants to achieve with the interaction: • Asks open-ended questions • Speaks directly to person with symptoms whenever possible • Listens attentively and interjects appropriately • Quantifies and qualifies symptoms (e.g., pain scales, pea size, quarter size, etc.) • Interprets the caller/patient's description of symptoms (location, appearance, etc.) • Repeats and clarifies caller/patient's statements for better understanding of descriptions • Identifies any hidden agendas for the call • Sorts and prioritizes symptoms • Is aware of self-diagnosis • Identifies primary and secondary symptoms • Focuses conversation for goal-directed, time-limited communication • Displays good speaking and writing skills	Uses effective interpersonal communication skills to engage in, develop, and disengage in a therapeutic interaction.

4. **Dimension: Telehealth Nursing Practice/Documentation**
Telehealth Standard V: Continuity of Care

Definition:
"Process of developing organized, integrated approaches to ensure that individuals and groups have timely, appropriate access to and utilization of health care services across the continuum of care" (AAACN, 2009, p. 33).
"Good documentation describes the nursing process of assessment, nursing diagnosis and planning, implementing, and evaluating patient care" (Espensen, 2009, p. 111).

Introduction:
The professional ambulatory care nurse documents patient encounters using standardized language in order to convey pertinent information to other providers and to ensure continuity of care throughout the health care system. Documentation serves to illustrate details of patient's current health status, relevant contributing factors, and rationale for disposition decisions. Documentation supports clinical decision-making, justifies billing, and may be used to defend in litigation situations.

Key Action Tips:
- Document both incoming and outgoing calls as they occur and communicate effectively with other team members to provide continuity of care and patient advocacy.
- Documentation should reflect nursing perspective of patient care by identifying assessment of patient and patient's perceived understanding of current health issues.

Example:
- Patient refuses to come in for clinic visit or present to ER; documentation should reflect nurse's attempt to identify barriers to care such as inability to procure transportation, other caregiver responsibilities, knowledge deficit, etc. Documentation should also include attempts to remedy refusal such as social work referral.
- Patient who is admitted following nursing telehealth encounter receives follow-up call after discharge from hospital to convey nurse's interest in patient outcomes and to provide continuity of care across the continuum.

Subtopic	Elements	Competency Statement
Telehealth Encounters	➤ Documentation reflects care and recommendations provided and includes: • Patient and record identifiers • Reason for the call • Complete assessment of the symptoms • Clinical guideline/protocol used for assessment and triage category • Comfort measures/home care provided • Allergies, current medications, medical history • Information and education provided • Disposition of patient; referrals provided or offered • Disclaimers given to the patient/caller • Patient's/caller's understanding of care plan of action, any refusal of care, and nurse's response to refusal • Reference sources used for care coordination ➤ Interventions completed ➤ Follow-up calls	Documents telecommunications that reflect care specific to the actual or potential health needs of the caller/patient.

5. Dimension: Personal/Professional Development

Definition:
"Accepts personal responsibility for maintaining and improving knowledge and skills necessary to assess, triage, and manage patients" (Laughlin, 2006, p. 144).

Introduction:
Professional development for nurses encompasses the journey from novice to expert. Nurses transitioning from inpatient to ambulatory care areas, while bringing valuable experiences, will need to develop new skills to manage patients using telehealth nursing principles.

Key Action Tips:
- The professional nurse develops awareness of personal, professional, and regulatory standards related to the delivery of patient care and assumes responsibility for continued competence.

Example:
- Adheres to continuing education requirements and maintains an unencumbered nursing license.
- Attends meetings of local, state, and (possibly) national nursing organizations.
- Networks with other nurses.
- Maintains membership in professional organizations such as AAACN.
- Seeks specialty certifications in ambulatory care nursing.
- Shares knowledge with others and mentors less-experienced nurses.

Subtopic	Elements	Competency Statement
Professional Development	➤ Demonstrates the commitment to enhance own clinical, telehealth, technical, medical, and legal knowledge for safe and effective nursing practice ➤ Readily attends all required education and competency programs directly related to practice area ➤ Initiates and participates in a wider variety of educational programs relevant to practice area, healthcare trends, and new clinical developments ➤ Articulates the value of telehealth nursing as related to improved patient outcomes ➤ Requests coaching and assistance from preceptors/other experienced staff when needed ➤ Willingly assists team members as needed ➤ Designs and presents unit education programs based on assessed needs of staff	Accepts personal responsibility for maintaining and improving the knowledge and skills necessary to assess, triage, and manage patients.

6. Dimension: Telehealth Nursing Practice/Resource Management

Definition:
"Resource management is an organization's ability to efficiently manage its resources, people, capital, equipment, and supplies" (Laughlin, 2006, p. 79).

Introduction:
Within the nursing profession, there are numerous opportunities to improve care while implementing cost-saving measures. Telehealth nursing is, in essence, a more cost-effective means to provide assessment and triage of patients.

Key Action Tips:
- The professional nurse is cognizant of the cost of care provided and seeks to minimize expenses through processes of delegation, judicious use of resources, and awareness of billing procedures and budgetary constraints.

Example:
- Seeks most economical means to provide excellent care by utilizing community support agencies and providing patient education to enable patient access to assistance.
- Delegates clerical and non-nursing tasks to assistive personnel.
- Develops awareness of cost of in-home assessment by visiting nurse vs. clinic visit vs. ER.
- Uses technology to streamline work and to avoid unnecessary repetitive tasks by the use of documentation templates.

Subtopic	Elements	Competency Statement
Internal and External Resource Utilization	➤ Identifies options and uses resources that relate to nursing practice and care: • Follows organization-defined procedures for managing a symptom-based call when no triage guideline is included in the clinical database • Accesses approved Internet sites to provide information • References sources of all information given outside of triage guidelines • Utilizes clinical assessment of caller variables to maintain appropriateness of disposition (defined urgency) with availability of clinical services (provider office, urgent care, ED, etc.) • Uses additional references when needed to provide caller/patient information • Schedules call-backs for callers as defined by need and/or policy	Locates and utilizes appropriate resources to meet the needs of the caller/patient.

7. Dimension: Telehealth Nursing Practice Issues
Telehealth Standard VI: Ethics & Patients' Rights

Definition:
"Professional ambulatory care nurses recognize the dignity, diversity, and worth of individuals and families, respect individual, cultural, spiritual, and psychosocial differences; and apply philosophical and ethical concepts that promote access to care, equality, and continuity of care" (AAACN, 2007, p. 13).

Introduction:
The nurse develops an awareness of cultural differences and adapts care to accommodate diverse populations and to overcome language barriers.

Key Action Tips:
- Provide culturally sensitive care.
- Provide referrals for mental health, abuse counseling, and other assessments if indicated.

Example:
- Utilizes interpreter services for patient communications.
- Protects personal health information and patients' rights to privacy.
- Nurse in the role of patient advocate.

Subtopic	Elements	Competency Statement
Issues	➤ Complies with department and organizational policies and procedures ➤ Manages emergency medical system or crisis intervention referrals ➤ Practices in a fair, non-discriminating way, acknowledging the difference in beliefs and cultural practice of callers/patients ➤ Maintains patient confidentiality and privacy during telehealth encounters ➤ Adheres to mandated reporting policies ➤ Contributes to caller/patient safety by ensuring a safe consultation through the use of established risk management procedures ➤ Comprehends and understands legislation, health, and social policy relevant to nursing practice ➤ Refrains from providing a diagnosis or giving personal opinions or advice ➤ Undertakes and records an accurate, thorough nursing assessment per the use of guidelines of the telehealth encounter	Practices in accordance with ethical, legal, and organizational framework that ensures the caller/patient's interest and well-being are met.

Telehealth Nursing Practice Orientation Competencies

Employee: _____ **Hire Date:** _____ **Preceptor:** _____

Orientation Competencies	Novice/Expert Weight Factor	Tested	Observed	Exceeds Expectations	Meets Expectations	Does Not Meet Expectations

Complies with call management standards:

1. Answers phone on or before 3 rings for ≥ 85% of all calls handled.
2. Responds to highest priority call in queue.
3. Call back to caller leaving message within 30 minutes for ≥ 85% of all calls handled.
4. Maintains professional composure in high-stress, emotional situations.
5. Maintains confidentiality of all interactions.
6. Manages ≥ 85% of population specific calls within the LOC benchmarks established by call center.

Source: Becker, 1999.

References

American Academy of Ambulatory Care Nursing (AAACN). (2007). *Telehealth nursing practice administration and practice standards* (4th ed.). Pitman, NJ: Author.

American Academy of Ambulatory Care Nursing (AAACN). (2009). *Ambulatory care nursing certification review course syllabus.* Pitman, NJ: Author.

Becker, C. (1999). *Telehealth nursing practice orientation competencies.* Unpublished manuscript.

Canadian Nurses Association (CNA). (2000). Telehealth: Great potential or risky terrain? *Nursing Now: Issues and Trends in Canadian Nursing, 9,* 1-4. Retrieved from http://cna-aiic.ca/cna/documents/pdf/publications/Telehealth_November2000_e.pdf

Espensen, M. (Ed). (2009). *Telehealth nursing practice essentials.* Pitman, NJ: American Academy of Ambulatory Care Nursing.

Laughlin, C.B. (Ed). (2006). *Core curriculum for ambulatory care nursing* (2nd ed.). Pitman, NJ: American Academy of Ambulatory Care Nursing.

Williams, C. (2008). Telehealth trials & triumphs: The self-diagnosed patient. *ViewPoint, 30*(2), 10-11.

Additional Readings

American Telemedicine Association. (2008). *Telehealth nursing.* A white paper developed and accepted by the Telehealth Nursing Special Interest Group.

Canadian Nurses Association (CNA). (2001). *The role of the nurse in telepractice.* Ottawa, ON: Author.

Melnyk, B.M. (2008). The latest evidence on telehealth interventions to improve patient outcomes. *Worldviews on Evidence-Based Nursing* (Third Quarter).

Swan, B., Conway-Phillips, R., & Griffin, K. (2006). Demonstrating the value of the RN in ambulatory care. *Nursing Economic$, 24*(6), 315-322.

Wright, D. (1998). *The ultimate guide to competency assessment in healthcare* (2nd ed.). Eau Claire, WI: Professional Education Systems, Inc.

Resources

Cleveland Clinic Foundation Nurse on Call, The. (n.d.). *Telehealth nursing practice call monitoring competency assessment tool.*

John A. Hartford Foundation Institute for Geriatric Nursing, The. (n.d.). *Ambulatory care GERO competencies.*

University of Michigan, The. (n.d.). *Competency program guidelines.*

Introduction to Ambulatory Care Staff Educator Competencies

Lenora J. Flint, MSN, MS, RN, PHN, CNS

The American Academy of Ambulatory Care Nursing defines *competence* as the ability to demonstrate the technical, critical thinking, and interpersonal skills necessary to perform one's job responsibly, including that of ambulatory care staff educators (Laughlin, 2006, p. 419). This definition is not stagnant; it embodies progress and advancement.

Ambulatory healthcare systems and resources continue to evolve over time to meet the ever-changing medical environment and demands placed upon it. Similarly, the role of the ambulatory care educator requires an ongoing and progressive shift in thinking, practice, and competence. Initiating, leading, and responding to healthcare challenges through the acquisition of knowledge and development of systems, processes, and skill sets are fundamental nursing attributes consistently demonstrated throughout its history. As you review the following examples of nursing education and educator milestones, consider the competency definition and your role as an ambulatory care staff educator or your perception of the role. Ask yourself: what has transformed and how has it influenced the role, responsibilities, and competence domain of the ambulatory care staff educator presently?

Florence Nightingale initiated staff development programs during the Crimean War (1854-1856) to improve the adequacy of nursing care for allied troops (Avillion, 2005). Following the war, she founded nurse training schools and developed standards to improve hospital care and efficiency. Additionally, Florence advocated for nursing education by modeling continuing learning and integration of knowledge, conducting research and employing data, coupled with astute political savvy and consultation skills to improve patient care outcomes.

Although the development of formal training nursing schools was prevalent during the late 1800s and early 1900s, several pioneers advocating staff development and ongoing continuation began publishing articles on the topic in nursing journals. Edna L. Foley, superintendent of the Visiting Nurses' Association in Chicago in 1912, proposed graduate nurses attend in-services and continuing education programs. In 1928, Blanche Pfefferkorn, executive secretary for the National League of Nursing, wrote a historical review of in-service education encouraging its expansion based upon the increasing complexity of nursing services and demands by hospitals for improvement of nursing schools and the quality of its graduates.

Historically, private duty nursing conducted in the patient's home was the common service setting; however, during the Great Depression in the late 1920s and 1930s, families ceased their ability to pay for home nursing care, resulting in many nurses returning to hospitals for work. This transition required re-orientation to the hospital environment and increased the demand and necessity for in-service training and on the job skill development; however, staff development departments did not exist and the responsibility for training the nurses was relegated to head nurses and supervisors.

During World War II (WWII), the new regime of hospital-trained nurses joined armed forces. Hospitals compensated for the RN shortage by hiring and training non-professional staff to assume former nursing duties which could be legally delegated to them. Staff educators' roles and responsibilities shifted accordingly to orienting and training support staff. Following WWII, medical technology and the advent of critical care units exploded, with subsequent opportunities and staff development needs for what was then referred to as *advanced nursing practice*. These milestones, accompanied by three entry levels of nursing (educational preparation diploma, associate, and baccalaureate degree), spurred the need for staff development to reinvent itself again. Orientation, in-service, and continuing education began to be viewed as requisite priorities by professional nursing organizations.

Between 1940 and 1960, staff education was the essential entity to train nurses on the proliferation of technological medical advances experienced during this period. In 1953, the Joint Commission for the Improvement of Care of the Patient (precursor of The Joint Commission) proposed the development of a department specifically devoted to the training and continuing education needs of nursing staff. Staff development was consequently propelled into and acknowledged as a specialty service. In 1969, the first national conference on continuing education for nurses was sponsored by the Medical College of Virginia's Health Sciences Division of Virginia Commonwealth University.

In the 1970s and 1980s, several staff development publications and national associations served to further promote staff development and continuing education as a specialty. Among them, the *Journal of Continuing Education in Nursing* was first published in 1973. The Council of Continuing Education was established by The American Nurses Association in 1973, followed by the *Guidelines for Staff Development* in 1978. In 1985, *The Journal of Nursing Staff Development* (now known as the *Journal for Nurses in Staff Development*) began publication. During this epoch, the women's movement and healthcare's acknowledgement as a business occurred, accompanied by a decrease in nursing enrollment, a shortage of working RNs, and yet another cycle of increased hiring and utilization of non-professional staff. Creative and aggressive recruitment of nurses who had not been actively employed in nursing generated a proliferation of RN refresher courses, business acumen programs, and recommencement of education and training for non-professionals by staff development.

Rapid advances in technology continued in the 1990s, accompanied by a focus on disease prevention and treatment in the storm of Acquired Immune Deficiency Syndrome (AIDS). Health care conglomerates, the introduction of diagnostic related groups (DRGs), health maintenance influences, proliferation of ambulatory, and long-term care facilities all surfaced to reduce length of hospital stays and the types of treatments. *Fiscal savvy* and *cost reduction* became the norm for healthcare organization survival. The venerated yet trepidation buzz word of this era was "downsizing." Healthcare personnel experienced layoffs with the first round of "cuts" frequently engulfing staff development departments. Validating the staff development's value to the organization's mission and bottom line utilizing data and outcomes became paramount. Creative strategies to "stay alive" surfaced with staff educators coordinating hospital-wide education as opposed to department-, task-, or discipline-specific training. New appellations, for example, *researcher, performance coach,* and *consultant,* supplemented the staff educator's roles and responsibilities. Staff development departments assumed new aliases, *professional development, organization development,* and *education and training center.* Qualifications for staff developers underscored management experience in contrast to clinical adeptness.

Notwithstanding the aforementioned challenges, in 1992, the ANA published *Roles and Responsibilities for Nursing Continuing Education and Staff Development Across All Settings,* nationally recognizing staff development's position as a healthcare and nursing stratagem and providing a systematic definition and structure for the specialty. Additionally in 1992, the first certification examination for nursing continuing education and staff development was inaugurated by The American Nurses Credentialing Center (ANCC). Both events served to demonstrate nurses' resilience and staying power in the ever-evolving healthcare arena.

Existing 21st century trends continue to affect and shape ambulatory care and nursing practice (for example, environmental threats, new emerging diseases, and increased aging population with ensuing increase in chronic diseases). Health care remains beneficiary to spiraling legislation and regulation with the Health Insurance Portability and Accountability Act (HIPAA), a notable example, mandating policy and procedures to secure personal health information (PHI). Additionally, exemplary customer service and accountability to consumers through systems structured to provide ethical clinical practice and business decisions are crucial to an organization's viability. These ever-changing supply and demand complexities continue to require new nursing knowledge and skill sets which reside within the purview of ambulatory staff development departments and educators.

Today's ambulatory care staff educators remain committed to providing outcomes that generate quality nursing services; however, informal feedback obtained at the AAACN national meeting in 2007 from individuals participating in the special interest staff development group (SIG), revealed the following concerns and experiences:

- Diminishing quantity of educators
- Dissolution of formal staff development departments
- Serving dual roles (e.g., department manager and "default staff educator")
- Lack of formal training as a staff educator
- Staff educator assignments situated far and wide, sometimes traveling up to 100 miles one way to provide education and training
- Orientation, training, and competence evaluation for predominantly clerical and support staff
- Emphasis on completing a mandatory education task as opposed to staff competence
- Annual versus ongoing competence assessment
- Department administrators holding staff educators totally accountable for staff competence
- A perception of the staff educator's role as "not valued"
- Minimal opportunities for research and professional networking
- Lack of knowledge and access to ambulatory care staff development resources and tools
- Joined AAACN and the Staff Ed SIG membership to network, obtain mentorship, educator job descriptions, competencies, and other adjuncts and training to assist them in becoming effective staff developers

The aforementioned concerns and current healthcare trends indicate ambulatory care educators simply cannot approach their duties as they have previously. Resources, tools, and collegial support must be harnessed to assist this nursing discipline and specialty to continue to meet challenges and equally add "value" to healthcare organizations. The staff educator competencies included in this edition of *Ambulatory Care Nursing Orientation and Competency Assessment Guide* is an initial response to support the dynamic role and responsibilities of those accountable for ambulatory care staff development.

References

Avillion, A.E. (2005). *Nurse educator manual: Essential skills and guidelines for effective practice.* Marblehead, MA: HCPro, Inc.

Laughlin, C.B. (Ed.). (2006). *Core curriculum for ambulatory care nursing* (2nd ed.). Pitman, NJ: American Academy of Ambulatory Care Nursing.

Chapter 6

Core Role Dimensions of an Ambulatory Care Staff Educator

Lenora J. Flint, MSN, MS, RN, PHN, CNS

Staff development is the process of providing continuing education and training for people working in organizations that specialize in the delivery of healthcare products and services (Avillion, 2005).

Introduction

Leader, facilitator, change agent, researcher, educator, and consultant are the six roles of an educator identified by the American Nurses Association (ANA, 2008). These roles are embedded in every aspect of ambulatory staff educator responsibilities. Whether teaching a class, planning an educational initiative, conducting research, serving on a committee, or conducting performance improvement activities, ambulatory staff educators have unequalled opportunity at every point of contact to demonstrate the value of education and the role of the educators to organizations and key stakeholders through consummate leadership, organizational visibility, and consultation. To demonstrate value, one must be competent and effectively articulate staff educator roles through actions and outcomes parallel to the mission, goals, and objectives of organizations. A commitment to continuing competence mandates lifelong learning activities for all professional nurses (ANA, 2008), including ambulatory staff educators.

Scenario: Repeat Blood Pressure Monitoring

Robin has been an ambulatory staff educator for three years. Her organization has established a 95% target for staff compliance in taking repeat blood pressures for patients with an elevated initial blood pressure reading during an ambulatory appointment. The electronic medical record "fires" an alert to direct the staff to take a repeat blood pressure. Performance improvement data reflects five of the six modules are below 70% compliance, with the remaining module at 89%. Although Robin had prior access and knowledge of the data, she recently was formally contacted by administration to fix the problem.

Review the scenario and complete the following:
1. List the staff educator competence skill set Robin needs to achieve her assignment.
2. Using the nursing process, draft an action plan integrating the skill sets you identified for Robin.
3. Describe how Robin can link her interventions and outcomes to patient safety.

Consider the following pearls as you read through the chapter:
- "The task of the modern educator is not to cut down jungles, but to irrigate deserts" (Lewis, 2007).
- "Leaders (educators) in ambulatory care need to spot toxic situations and initiate proactive steps to resolve them" (Swanson, 2006).
- Strategic plans evaluate the organization and help it attain long-term goals and objectives (Swanson, 2006).
- Planning, execution, and behaviors must remain aligned with the organization's ambitions.
- Staff educators retain accountability to influence the care agenda through modeling, communication, and consultation.
- The consultant role is critical to shaping the future of professional nursing through other nurses by enabling them to develop their practice.
- Staff educators are economically vital adjuncts to healthcare.
- Value through measurable outcomes is fundamental to quality ambulatory healthcare.

Core Role Dimension	Elements	Competency Statement
Customer Service	➤ Program strategic planning ➤ Resource management; human and financial ➤ Collaboration ➤ Teamwork/teambuilding ➤ Professional networking ➤ Prioritization of needs and plans to achieve goals ➤ Systematic problem-solving ➤ Advocacy for ambulatory care as a specialty ➤ Change agent ➤ Ethical integrity	Proactively charts an education and competency pathway that supports the organization's values through development and preservation of "state of the art" staff competence.
Organizational Visibility	➤ Competent staff ➤ Achieved outcomes ➤ Marketing ➤ Communication ➤ Role model ➤ Active committee membership ➤ Systems and process improvements	Quantifies outcomes and provides ongoing communication and data to leaders and key stakeholders that delineate the staff educator's value to the organization's economic, social, and political agenda.
Consultant	➤ Expert practice ➤ Problem identification and resolution ➤ Coach ➤ Transformational leadership ➤ Emancipatory techniques ➤ Research and evaluation ➤ Learning culture	Demonstrates resourcefulness by counseling and guiding leadership, key stakeholders, and staff on initiatives to improve healthcare services and quality clinical outcomes.

I. Leader

A *leader* is not dependent on a title or formal authority; a leader is anyone who influences a group of people towards a specific result. Leaders demonstrate persistence and risk taking. *Leadership* is one of the most relevant aspects of the organizational context. Leadership is using one's influence to obtain assistance and support of others to achieve a task. Effective leadership is the ability to successfully integrate and maximize available resources within the internal and external environment to achieve organizational or societal goals.

Leaders in organizations engage *strategic planning* as a means to define its direction and chart its future course. Planning delineates quantifiable goals and objectives, and allocates resources including capital and people. Organizations derive and correlate the strategic plan to their mission and vision statements. A mission statement describes the fundamental purpose of the organization. It defines the customer and the essential processes and conveys the desired level of performance. The vision statement is source of motivation, explaining what the organization wants to be and provides clear decision-making criteria. A strategic plan usually answers one or all of the following questions: what is it that we do, who do we do it for (mission), and how can we excel (vision)? The organization's response to the aforementioned questions helps determine where it is presently, where it wants to go, how it will get there, and how it will know it has arrived there. The resulting document is referred to as the *strategic plan*. Collectively, the organization's mission, vision, and strategic plan are the framework used by savvy staff educators to develop actionable education goals and objectives.

A central component of staff educator responsibilities is developing strategies supported by quantifiable and achievable goals that synchronize with the bottom-line of organizations. Effective strategies include prudent management of both financial and human resources (Swanson, 2006). Educators can position themselves as contributing leaders to the organization by developing productive relationships with administration and key stakeholders. Competent communication, problem-solving, negotiation skills, and ongoing evaluation of educational program effectiveness (including financial management) are premier aspects of staff educators' program strategic planning. These value behaviors promote organizational visibility and lend themselves favorably to the inclusion of educators on prominent leader and decision-making committees.

Scenario: Repeat Blood Pressure Monitoring

The literature is replete in identifying the economic burden of chronic conditions. In 1996, almost half of the U.S. health care cost, $62.3 billion, was borne by one-quarter of the population with one or more of the following five conditions: mood disorders, diabetes, heart disease, asthma, and hypertension (Druss & Marcus, 2001).

Identify the proactive leadership opportunity Robin initially overlooked.

1. What strategies can Robin utilize to keep administration and other key stakeholders apprised of her action plan and outcomes to enhance her leadership visibility as a contributor to the organization's strategic plan?
2. What financial and human resources does Robin need to draw upon to accomplish her assignment?
3. Identify the mission, vision, and strategic plans for the organization in which you work.
4. How well does your staff educator annual plan equate to your organization's mission, vision, and strategic plan?

Collaboration is the process of healthcare professionals and stakeholders working toward a common goal by sharing knowledge, learning, and building consensus. Structured collaboration promotes introspection and acknowledgement of the benefits and shortfalls individual members bring to the team as a whole towards goal achievement. A team that works in partnership benefits from united resources in lieu of limited assets and can develop strong alliances. The staff educator's affiliation with work teams, including administration and key stakeholders, requires skilled leadership and effective communication skills to build and maintain dynamic professional rapport essential to achieve seamless healthcare services.

In the book *Crossing the Quality Chasm*, the Institute of Medicine (IOM, 2001) indicated improvement of the quality of healthcare collaboration among healthcare teams is essential to meet the demands of new technology, payers, and the healthcare environment at large. Post publication summit findings stated healthcare professionals were not adequately prepared to provide the highest quality and safest medical care possible, and inadequate assessment of their clinical competency exists. Additional findings noted that despite change made through the years, the basic approach to clinical education has not varied since 1910. They went on to recommend educators and others be held to assess and restructure clinical education for all healthcare professionals (including staff educators) to maintain staff proficiency in five core areas:

1. Work as part of an interdisciplinary team (collaboration)
2. Deliver patient-centered care
3. Practice evidence-based care
4. Focus on quality improvement
5. Use information technology

Multiple staff educators on a team are not always the best solution for resolving issues that appear to have an "education" premise. Sheer supply and demand of educators necessitates creative options. Collaborative techniques and teams can aptly assist educators to optimize benefits and minimize duplication of services, unachievable as a singular entity. Through program design and partnership with nurse managers, supervisors, preceptors, validators, and technology, educators can more effectively reach staff at large. In 2004, a review of the literature on interdisciplinary collaboration (Horak, Pauig, Keidan, & Kerns, 2004) demonstrated a significant relationship exists between enhanced team interactions, compliance, and improved clinical outcomes. Direct input from front line staff strengthens the educator's strategic plans and outcomes. Prudent utilization of staff adds worth and contributes to the success of the educator.

Scenario: Repeat Blood Pressure Monitoring

Take a moment to review the initial scenario and the action plan you developed for Robin to successfully complete her assignment.

1. Does your action plan include the five core areas recommended by the summit?
2. What information technology and processes could prove beneficial to the work team?

Collaboration and teamwork are concomitant. *Teamwork* is a joint action by two or more people in which each person contributes their talents, skill set, interests, and opinions to unify the group to achieve a common goal. While diversity in teams is recognized and celebrated as a value asset, teamwork is most effective when all participants harness and harmonize their forte working toward a universal aim. Teamwork does not mean individualism is no longer valued; it denotes efficient teamwork extends beyond individual accomplishments, with team players subordinating their personal aspirations for the betterment of the whole.

A staff educator competent in teambuilding facilitates teams in transitioning through the forming, storming, norming, and performing stages typically experienced by work teams. Inspiration, directing, delegating, supporting, coaching empowerment, and recognition and reward are examples of team management strategies utilized by the educator to develop participants' ability to work adeptly as a group. These strategies also include helping participants identify and alleviate impediments. Venerated deliverables from able healthcare teams consist of positive morale, improved communication and problem-solving, seamless care coordination, enhanced competence, and increased productivity and enhanced patient safety outcomes.

Scenario: Repeat Blood Pressure Monitoring
1. What disciplines do you suggest Robin include and collaborate with on her work team and why?
2. Outline an agenda for Robin to use in her first meeting with the team which could assist in unifying the group.
3. What handout material should Robin package to serve as a point of reference for team members?
4. Consider your facility. In addition to achieving the outcome goal of 95% compliance for taking a repeat blood pressure, what associated clinical and team quality improvement opportunities exist?

Professional networking is a process of building professional relationships through interactions with others who have common interest or goals. It involves getting to know other people and exchanging talents, expertise, and interests with the expectation that mutual benefits and assistance may transpire. Tapping into and expanding one's networking skills is a vital and rewarding component of staff educators' professional development. Within today's healthcare realm of limited and competitive resources, coupled with increasing demands and abridged deadlines, knowing the right people can strengthen staff educators' ability to get things done quickly and productively. Additionally, interactions with other educators can serve to validate one's practice and provide new ways of looking at situations, stimulating creativity and improving effectiveness of the educational process (Johnson, 2006).

Professional organizations generate standards of practice and proffer education, research, publishing, and volunteer opportunities. Active participation in a professional organization promotes networking with peers from a wide geographical area. Examples of AAACN's networking vehicles include an annual national conference with expert presenters, organization Web site with invaluable publications and resources, expert panel to pose questions and obtain recommendations, reference books, live audio

seminars, corporate collaborations, education courses, and special interest groups, one of which is the staff educator group. Additionally, training, tools, and resources for acquisition of specialty certification are available, which brings stature to the educator role. Staff educators must continually and proactively increase their array of internal, external, local, state, and national contacts to elevate and augment their practice. Doing so favorably serves to set them apart from the competition through expansion of one's professional profile and reputation.

Scenario: Repeat Blood Pressure Monitoring
1. Explain how Robin can utilize networking techniques to promote teambuilding and teamwork.
2. Additionally, identify the systems and processes Robin can "tap" to obtain evidenced-based practice data specific to blood pressure monitoring and hypertension.

Prioritizing needs and plans to achieve goals are equal key components of the educator's skill set. Maintaining preferential focus on the mission, vision, and values of the organization promotes their integration as core guiding principles in planning educational programs. Day-to-day competing activities and demands can cloud the educator's perception of what is important. It is easy to fall prey to reacting to an event instead of taking a broader look at the situation and conducting a root-cause analysis. A systems approach to problem-solving helps keep organizational goals at the forefront. Educators must think vertically as well as laterally, considering the whole and understanding how all the parts (including their role and responsibilities) work together. Prioritizing a need or part of a plan should always have the end product or goal taken into consideration (Coonan, 2007). A competent educator is knowledgeable with terms and metrics commonly used to discern their priority contribution. Linking metrics that drive organizations, staff competency, controlling high blood pressure, customer service, and member satisfaction for example, to the staff educator role, education plan, interventions, and outcomes not only demonstrates priority management and quality, but highlights value as well.

Staff educators as leaders are expected to prioritize and resolve a wide array of problems that are embedded in everyday practice and span from simplistic to complex. *Systemic problem-solving* is a mental process that draws upon one's knowledge, facts, principles, and cognitive ability to solve unknown problems. A systematic way to think through a problem to formulate objective options based upon data, experience, and reasonableness is referred to as a *train of thought*. Problem-solving, critical thinking, and decision-making are inseparable. The literature is replete with varied problem-solving tools and techniques that range from basic to very sophisticated. Common tools familiar to most educators include

Nursing Process	Purpose	Reframed Common Problem-Solving Approach Steps
Assessment	➤ Assess situation ➤ Systematic approach to assess situation ➤ Obtain subjective and objective data ➤ Verify and organize data ➤ Triage and prioritize data	Describe the problem.
Diagnosis	➤ Analyzes data ➤ Defines the problem ➤ Diagnosis provides clinical direction	Analyze the cause.
Planning	➤ Defines specific action for achieving goals and desired outcomes that guide the implementation process ➤ Establishes realistic goals that are objective, realistic, and measurable	Identify and assess options.
Implementation	➤ Individualized priority actions performed to achieve specified goal	Choose one option and implement it.
Evaluation	➤ Assessment of response and degree of response to plan of care ➤ Reassessment or re-planning	Evaluate outcomes.

brainstorming, root analysis, research, networking, and cause and effect analysis, but too often we overlook utilization of the nursing process. While an array of problem-solving approaches exist, most are generally comprised of all or part of the nursing process, a systematic framework promoting critical thinking and decision-making. Staff educators are encouraged to consider the nursing process framework as they problem-solve and lead others to resolve daily challenges.

Scenario: Repeat Blood Pressure Monitoring

1. Re-examine the action plan you developed for Robin. Does it correlate to the five steps of the nursing process framework? If not, what's missing in your action plan?
2. What priority metrics did you include in the action plan you developed for Robin? Are they relevant and quantifiable?

An ongoing challenge of ambulatory care nursing is its acknowledgement as a specialty. To this aim, AAACN has identified advocacy as one of its goals; nurses, employers, and third party payers will recognize and value ambulatory care nursing. Advocacy is the proactive process of addressing issues of concern to wield influence on behalf of people, or a concept to bring about social, political, and economic changes. Florence Nightingale thrived as an activist and utilized her talents to reform the world at large even when she became an invalid. Without setting one foot in India, she intervened in its politics, chastising her government for periodic famines that took the lives of 20 million people during British rule (Hanink, 2009). Similarly, ambulatory staff educators reside in tactical positions to articulate the difference between nurses' roles in the ambulatory and inpatient setting, using variables identified by AAACN to distinguish and promote ambulatory care nursing as a specialty. The distinctions between nurse practice in the inpatient setting and that of ambulatory care are generally not recognized and appreciated by healthcare organizations. Staff educators must exert every opportunity to convey the distinctions to embody a mutual respect and esteem for the unique characteristics of each entity and their role and contributions within the context of healthcare. Both entities are invaluable. The educator's ability to articulate ambulatory care's fundamental mission, vision, goals and objectives, and supporting systems and processes, including staff skill set, is requisite for advocacy. Active membership in AAACN, submersion in its functions, tapping into its available resources, and networking are invaluable toward this end. Educators as leaders retain accountability to influence the care agenda through modeling, communication, organizational visibility, and consultation.

Scenario: Repeat Blood Pressure Monitoring

1. What opportunities are available for Robin to advocate for ambulatory care nursing as a specialty in the project she has been assigned? Be specific.
2. What benefits could Robin receive to assist her advocacy for ambulatory nursing at her facility by being an active member AAACN?

Advocacy, a staff educator role element, is allied with the change agent function. A *change agent* is someone that brings about, or helps bring about change by assisting people to increase their productivity and quality of services. A change agent is self-motivated, future oriented, goal-driven, passionate, and inspires and understands others. Although the definition may sound lofty, change is not to be underestimated. It is hard work. Change removes us from our comfort zone and does not always yield the intended results. Additionally, change requires the staff educator to call upon a wide-range of skill depending upon the task at hand. Staff educator skill sets elicited will be dictated by the dimensions of the projected change process (for example, resources, timeframe, end goal, and mutual acceptance of change process) by change participants and recipients. Assisting the organization to meet the 95% compliance target for staff repeating blood pressures after an alert is triggered in the electronic record requires a different skill set than providing basic life support classes. Although there is no "ideal" change agent, a staff educator's change agent competencies can have a major effect on the success or failure of a project. Buchanan and Boddy (1992) identified fifteen "key" competencies of effective change agents:

1. Sensitivity to how change impacts key personnel, including top management's perception and how these perceptions may impact the project goals
2. Establishment of clear, defined, quantifiable, and realistic goals
3. Flexibility in response to change with corresponding change in management style
4. Teambuilding capability with the inclusion of key stakeholders and delegation of responsibility
5. Networking
6. Ambiguity tolerance
7. Effective communication across all levels of healthcare providers
8. Interpersonal skills
9. Enthusiasm for project
10. People motivator
11. Successful marketing of plans that defines the vision and obtains buy-in
12. Negotiation and conflict management skills to overcome barriers and obtain project resources
13. Political astuteness
14. Influencing skills
15. Ability to see the "big" picture and not just the immediate project

Change within the healthcare system is prolific as witnessed by the flux of healthcare legislation, new care initiatives, national quality metrics, evidence-based practice, and advanced technology. The staff educator in ambulatory care cannot be complacent or content with the status quo and expect to add value. Change is probably the only constant. Organizations expect staff educators to be proactive leaders at the forefront to assist in sustaining their viability.

Scenario: Repeat Blood Pressure Monitoring

1. Which of the fifteen competencies identified by Buchanan and Boddy (1992) would prove most beneficial for Robin to be competent with to successfully complete the project she been assigned and why?

2. What negative symbolisms may occur if Robin is unsuccessful with the assigned project?
3. Which of the fifteen competencies have you engaged in a current project to which you are assigned in your facility? Which competencies did you not use and why?

Nurse ethic refers to what we ought to reasonably do and how we ought to act in a given situation (Gold, 2006). Ethics incorporates standards relating to rights that benefit society, requiring staff educators to continuously examine their own moral beliefs and conduct to assure they live up to standards that are reasonable and sound within the context of their practice domain and the organizations they help shape. *Integrity* is unwavering ownership and observance to high moral and ethical principles or professional standards. Integrity requires three steps: (1) discerning what is right and what is wrong; (2) acting on what you have discerned even at personal cost; and (3) saying openly that you are acting on your understanding of right from wrong (Carter, 1996). Individuals who have *ethical integrity* base everything that they do and believe on a core set of values.

Ethical integrity and its principles serve a foundation that stabilizes nursing practice in the midst of constant change to secure society's trust in the profession. The practice of nursing professional development is guided by principles of ethics (ANA, 2005). Each state's registered nurse practice act also identifies duty owed to consumers. The ANA code of ethics for nurses prescriptively delineates nurses' obligations to:

- Respect the dignity of the individual, whatever the socioeconomic status, personal attributes, or type of health problem
- Safeguard the patient's right to confidentiality
- Protect the patient and public from unsafe or unethical practices
- Exercise responsibility and accountability for nursing actions
- Maintain own practice competencies
- Exercise professional knowledge and judgment in accepting and carrying out assignments and in delegating to others (ANA, 2008)

Ethical integrity is measured through compliance to the following principles that guide ethical decision-making (Gold, 2006):

- Autonomy: self-determination; the ability to exercise and choose and make one's own decisions without coercion
- Beneficence: doing good by conducting that which is in the patient's best interest
- Non-malfeasance: avoiding intentional or unintentional harm
- Justice: equitable distribution and use of resources
- Veracity: truth telling

- Confidentiality: proactively protecting the patient and family's privacy rights
- Fidelity: faithfully fulfilling duty to patients, family and colleagues, and self

Ethical standards and principles are not limited to the ambulatory clinical practice arena, but are inclusive of staff educator roles and responsibility within their practice setting. Staff educators must be cognitive of and competent in consistently role modeling ethical integrity. This can be achieved by taking advantage of every opportunity to continuously integrate the standards into the formal and informal interactions with staff. In addition to providing classroom training on ethical integrity, educators are encouraged to consistently weave ethical integrity principles and standards into all in-service offerings. For example, training on documentation, at minimum, should include the nurse practice act, evidence-based practice, the organization's documentation policies and procedures, and the Health Insurance Portability and Accountability Act (HIPAA). Following in-service training, staff educators must transition out of their offices and classrooms into the clinical arena to observe and reinforce staff adherence to these standards. Staff educators are also encouraged to actively participate on the organization's ethics committee.

Scenario: Repeat Blood Pressure Monitoring

1. During Robin's assessment of staff members and their compliance in conducting repeat blood pressures when a best practice alert "fires," she is privately notified by a staff member that a colleague "makes up" the numbers she records for repeat blood pressures. How, if at all, should Robin proceed?
2. How do you measure staff compliance with ethical integrity within your scope of responsibilities as an educator at your facility?

II. Organizational Visibility

Participation on essential internal and external committees is one of several ways staff educators can market their organizational visibility. Additional methods include assuring competent staff; demonstrating quantifiable outcomes that link directly to the organization's strategic plans; delivery of effective, timely, and relevant communication; professional role modeling; and ongoing systems and process improvements. Assertively integrating these and other visibility techniques to promote value of staff educators to the organizations is central to survival within the existing healthcare's economic climate. Too often the benefits of staff educators go unrecognized. Failure to consistently contribute to the organization's bottom line brings unwanted visibility of an expendable nature. Staff educators' indispensable assets must be consistently demonstrated through their behaviors and actions and generate a worthy, palpable, and enduring presence.

The Joint Commission and the Accreditation Association for Ambulatory Health Care provide accreditation for ambulatory care facilities. Both organizations have standards that require validation of staff competence, orientation to the organization, quality measure initiatives, and outcomes. Achievement of these standards is core to staff educator responsibilities, placing them in a pivotal position of power and influence. Educators must understand this power and influence and how best to maximize it to their "visibility" benefit. Organizational leaders and staff educators generally work together as a team to accomplish the education and quality initiatives, making it crucial for staff educators to maintain ongoing communication regarding their education program strategies, progress, and outcomes. It is not enough to report the number of classes and in-services provided to staff. Staff educators must provide granular data and action plans attuned to the language of organizational leaders by reporting outcomes that link to the overall facility goals, particularly patient safety. In this manner staff educators add value coupled with organizational visibility. Let's use Robin to illustrate these points further:

Staff compliance was scheduled by the organization as one of several steps determined to support the strategic plan of 5% improvement in hypertension control in patients over the preceding year. In support of this initiative, Robin utilized evidence-based guidelines and the organization's blood pressure monitoring procedure to educate and verify staff competency in taking blood pressures. She determined staff to be competent and reported 100% compliance with taking accurate blood pressure to leadership and administration.

However, during Robin's preliminary assessment of potential barriers to staff conducting a repeat blood pressure when warranted, she notices that an untoward percentage of staff are not adhering to the guidelines which include: patient sitting upright with their back supported, both feet on the floor, absence of talking, and the blood pressure arm supported at heart level. Additionally, she witnesses several staff placing the blood pressure cuff over heavy clothing. She is surprised as the individuals are the staff she approved as competent three months ago. Does this sound all too familiar? Robin appropriately engaged evidence-based guidelines in her in-services, as she is familiar with the fact that guidelines can significantly improve patient safety. What she failed to appreciate is data indicates guideline compliance tends to be low and varies from 20% to 100% (Gurses & Murphy, 2009). An equal culprit that educators need to be increasingly attentive to is their accountability in sustaining ongoing competence. In addition to reporting 100% compliance in monitoring blood pressures, Robin could increase her contributions and value by developing and sharing an action plan with key stakeholders to sustain compliance and thus patient safety. Competency is much more than a one-time annual achievement; it is an ongoing process.

A superlative job description can equally serve to promote staff educator visibility and assist leaders' understanding of the role and responsibilities of staff educators. However, a word of caution: these same leaders will expect and hold the educator accountable to meet the dimensions of the job description. Educators must be intimately familiar with their job description and review them at minimum annually to assure the job functions and competencies specified are pertinent, realistic, and achievable. Most importantly, the job description should align with the culture, goals, and future direction of the organization.

Staff educators must continually market themselves to the organization by participating in systems and process improvement initiatives. Staff educator roles inherently lend themselves to incorporation of evidence-based nurse practice. Competent staff educators remain current and in tune with "state of the art" practice standards and integrate research findings that improve nurse practice and patient outcomes in ambulatory care. Effective staff educators proactively seek more effective, efficient, and economical ways to keep staff competent and engaged in quality services which translate to organizational visibility and merit for nursing at large.

Consultant

All staff educators act in a formal or informal consultant role (ANA, 2008). A *consultant* is considered a content expert who has an expansive access to resources to specific subject matter. Consultants offer their skills to others, give advice, coach, identify problems and recommend resolution, provide training, or perform specialized work with the intent of improving outcomes. The educator consultant role is becoming more commonplace, given the complexities, challenges, and economics of the healthcare industry. With an emphasis on improving employee and patient satisfaction, many organizations recognize a need to change their culture. In the consultant role, the staff educator aspires to shape the environment and its resources towards outcomes that ensure efficient and effective patient care. Target outcomes for this role are to transform culture, develop evidenced-based practice, and promote patient-centered practice. Manley (2001) identified six core skills and qualities fundamental to the nurse consultant role:

1. Ability to apply the practice of nursing to a specific client group, whether as a generalist or a specialist
2. Leadership and strategic vision
3. Engage research and evaluation approaches that focus on day-to-day issues in practice
4. Facilitate practice development and structural, cultural, and practice change
5. Create a learning culture; one that enables all members of the interdisciplinary team to learn and develop their potential
6. Provide consultancy from a clinical level in relationship to individual patients, to organizational levels in terms of the provision of patient-centered services

An effective educator consultant is able to draw on three key processes which fall within the six core qualities and skills identified by Manley: transformational leadership, emancipatory methodologies, and practice expert. *Transformational leadership* is the process of developing staffs' leadership potential within a shared and common vision while *emancipatory* processes involve helping others to overcome barriers within themselves, their work flow, and work environment. Methods inclusive of emancipatory processes are action learning, one-to-one, and group clinical supervision through engagement of skilled facilitation. As a *practice expert*, one serves and is viewed as a role model. Additionally, a staff educator practice leader has an established track record of improving nursing practice and outcomes. A practice expert is intimately engaged in the daily core practice of others, rather than establishing discrete conditions such as "rounding" to demonstrate what can be achieved in daily practice. However, Manley (2002a) cautions that a consultant cannot afford to simply "do" practice. The doing must be accompanied by facilitation with staff to enable them to see and experience alternative ways of doing things. Everything the educator does in the consultant role must not only enable others to develop their practice, but must also help embed cultural changes in the workplace. Thus, an educator providing typical classroom or skill lab education and training will not be demonstrating the full potential and effectiveness of the consultant role. The expertise of a consultant educator resides in being able to facilitate others to change their practice culture. A paramount outcome for the educator consultant role is linking strategies to the practice setting (for example, enabling nurses to minimize patient gaps in care through systematic utilization of a patient healthcare database at each patient encounter).

The literature correlates the consultative role to leadership. The consultant role is about shifting practice related to a strategic plan. There is also evidence that the consultant role promotes the coordination of care services and fosters inter-professional working (Manley, 2002b). Staff educators serving in the consultant role must be able to explain the practice element of their role and demonstrate its organizational strategic focus and outcomes. Without such, there is a clear and present danger of compensating for ineffective or absent management or worse yet, undermining management. Clear roles and accountabilities must be developed to ensure others act and reinforce the plans extended by the educator consultant. Structured evaluation of the contributions and more importantly, effectiveness of the consultants' competence in developing strategies that affirmatively improve practice environment outcomes by key stakeholders, is essential to improve patient outcomes, teamwork, job satisfaction, and value.

Changing the way an organization works, communicates, thinks, behaves, and values is a daunting task. An educator consultant can provide guidance to direct cultural changes; however, when exacting the consultant role, one must understand that cultural changes run a protracted course. Effective consultation practices work collaboratively with the organization's leaders. Implementation is the culmination of the role, and operationalizing plans will go smoother if key stakeholders and staff are involved continually in the process. Effective consultants mentor, coach, and inspire change in addition to providing valid, corroborated data to benchmark change. Consultation strategies and interventions must be measured and evaluated with successes celebrated.

References

American Nurses Association (ANA). (2005). *Code of ethics for nurses.* Retrieved from http://www.nursingworld.org/MainMenuCategories/EthicsStandards/CodeofEthicsforNurses.aspx

American Nurses Association (ANA). (2008). *Scope and standards of practice for nursing professional development.* Washington, D.C.: Author.

Avillion, A.E. (2005). *Nurse educator manual: Essential skills and guidelines for effective practice.* Marblehead, MA: HCPro, Inc.

Buchanan, D., & Boddy, D. (1992). *The expertise of the change agent: Public performance and backstage activity.* Prentice Hall.

Carter, S.L. (1996). *Integrity.* New York: BasicBooks/HarperCollins.

Coonan, P. (2007). *A practical guide to leadership development skills for the nurse manager.* Marblehead, MA: HCPro, Inc.

Druss, B., & Marcus, S. (2001). Comparing the national economic burden of five chronic conditions. *Health Affairs, 20*(6), 233-241.

Gold, C. (2006). Ethics. In C.B. Laughlin (Ed.), *Core curriculum for ambulatory care nursing* (2nd ed., pp. 183-187). Pitman, NJ: American Academy of Ambulatory Care Nursing.

Gurses, A.P., & Murphy, D.J. (2009). A practical tool to identify and eliminate barriers to compliance with evidence-based guidelines. *The Joint Commission Journal on Quality and Patient Safety, 35*(10), 526-532, 485.

Hanink, E. (2009, May 4). Florence Nightingale, multilingual mathematician. *Working Nurse Magazine*, p. 30.

Horak, B.J., Pauig, J., Keidan, B., & Kerns, J. (2004). Patient safety: A case study in team building and interdisciplinary collaboration. *Journal for Healthcare Quality, 26*(2), 6-13.

Institute of Medicine (IOM). (2001). Crossing the quality chasm: A new health system for the 21st century. Washington, D.C.: National Academy Press.

Johnson, E.M. (2006). Advocacy. In C.B. Laughlin (Ed.), *Core curriculum for ambulatory care nursing* (2nd ed., pp. 117-124). Pitman, NJ: American Academy of Ambulatory Care Nursing.

Lewis, C.S. (2007). Quotes. In E. Gruwell (Ed.), *The gigantic book of teachers' wisdom.* New York: Skyhorse Publishing, Inc.

Manley, K. (2001). *Consultant nurse: Concept, processes, outcome* [Unpublished doctoral study]. University of Manchester/Consultant Nurse Institute London.

Manley, K. (2002a). Refining the consultant nurse framework: Commentary on critiques. *Nursing in Critical Care, 7*(2), 84-87.

Manley, K. (2002b, May). The consultant nurse role. *NHS Journal for Healthcare Professions*, pp. 8-9.

Swanson, J. (2006). Leadership. In C.B. Laughlin (Ed.), *Core curriculum for ambulatory care nursing* (2nd ed., pp. 153-161). Pitman, NJ: American Academy of Ambulatory Care Nursing.

Additional Readings

American Academy of Ambulatory Care Nursing (AAACN). (2010). *Scope and standards of practice for professional ambulatory care nursing* (8th ed.) Pitman, NJ: Author.

Blanchard, K. (1985). *Leadership and the one-minute manager.* New York: William Morrow and Company.

Brunt, B.A., Pack, J.T., & Parr, P. (2001). The history of staff development. In A.E. Avillion (Ed.), *Core curriculum for staff development* (2nd ed.). Pensacola, FL: National Nursing Staff Development Organization.

Carroll, P. (2006). *Nursing leadership and management: A practical guide.* Clifton Park, NY: Thomason/Delmar Learning.

D'Angelo, L. (2006). Healthcare fiscal management. In C.B. Laughlin (Ed.), *Core curriculum for ambulatory care nursing* (2nd ed., pp. 73-81). Pitman, NJ: American Academy of Ambulatory Care Nursing.

Dewing, J., & Reid, B. (2003). A model for clinical practice within the consultant nurse role. *Nursing Times, 99*(9). Retrieved from http://www.nursingtimes.net

Donahue, P.M. (1985). *Nursing: The finest art, an illustrated history.* St. Louis: The C.V. Mosby Company.

Gardner, J.W. (1989). The tasks of leadership. In W.E. Rosenbach & R.L. Taylor (Eds.), *Contemporary issues in leadership* (2nd ed., pp. 24-33). Boulder, CO: Westview Press.

Haas, S. (2006). Ambulatory care nursing specialty practice. In C.B. Laughlin (Ed.), *Core curriculum for ambulatory care nursing* (2nd ed., pp. 3-4). Pitman, NJ: American Academy of Ambulatory Care Nursing..

Nightingale, F. (1859). *Notes on nursing.* London: Harrison and Sons.

Chapter 7

Planning Education and Validation Programs

Donna Pforr, BSN, EdM
Maj Carla Leeseberg, USAF AFMOA, AFMOA/SGNE
Linda Brixey, RN

Knowing the needs and/or goals of the organization and those of the student are equally important. Conducting a needs assessment prior to program development can make the educator more effective. Knowing what topic the organization wants delivered and what the learning deficits of the staff are provides direction for educational initiatives. Learning is an interdependent process and is most effective when students construct their own meaning of knowledge (Huang, 2006, p. 31). Knowles' Adult Learning Theory focuses on the needs of the learner and on the learning being self-directed and teaching adults to be in control of their own learning (Mitchell & Courtney, 2005). The learning is facilitated by the educator using a variety of modes of delivery to meet their learning needs.

Analysis of findings from the needs assessment can allow the educator to distinguish competency issues versus performance issues. If the problem has its basis in the nurse's performance, education is unlikely to make a difference. In this case the nurse knows how to do the competency but chooses to take shortcuts or disregard proper procedure. This is a management issue, not an educational deficit. If the issue is based on a lack of knowledge, an educational program can make a difference by improving the nurse's understanding and competency.

Promoting competency-based practice is one of the methods educators may use to plan an effective educational program. *Competency-based practice (CBP)* is defined as a patient care delivery system that emphasizes the nurse's ability to demonstrate competence in the high-risk, high-volume, and problem-prone aspects of care related to a specific role and clinical setting. Unlike traditional nursing practice models, CBP expectations are derived from the "real world" of nursing and focus on *"doing"* rather than on only "knowing." A *competency statement* is a broad statement of expected performance. If, for example, when expected to care for patients with diabetes, a competency statement could be stated as "the nurse provides education, training, and support to meet the needs of diabetic patients with abnormal glycemic control."

When developing a program, always know the overall goal. From the goal, objectives are developed that define how learners will achieve the goal. The objectives, stated in measurable terms, are used to determine the content of the program. Some goals can be accomplished in a few objectives and in a short program. Others that are more extensive may require multiple goals, defined objectives, and multiple learning interventions over a period of time to be accomplished.

Key Points:

- Assessing needs and/or goals of the organization is a first step in building educational programs.
- Assessment of individual learning needs is considered in development of the content.
- Determine the goal of the program and objectives prior to content development.
- Plan what data to collect to demonstrate the effectiveness of education given.
- Use program evaluations to improve recurrent programs and to create new ones.

Example

A common colloquialism has been repeated over time in learning or teaching situations: "See one, do one, teach one." Behavior may be changed when there is opportunity to observe the right and wrong way to do something. If the nurse has learned something incorrectly or if the process has changed but extra care was not taken to implement the change, the nurse may not understand why the change is needed (cognitive ability). She may rely on past instruction and experience. Educators need to be cognizant of their own behavior and the tools used in programs they develop to create learning experiences for the student. An effective needs assessment will direct more accurate educational planning that meets the needs of the learner and organization goals.

Subtopic	Elements	Competency Statement
Needs Assessment – Initiates an Appraisal Process to Guide Program Development	➤ Incorporates the organization's mission, vision, values, and strategic plan ➤ Utilizes evidenced-based practice ➤ Complies with community standards ➤ Addresses the needs of program participants ➤ Demonstrates awareness of health care trends and reform ➤ Incorporates regulatory guidelines ➤ Can discuss community and societal needs ➤ Conforms to policy and procedures ➤ Participates in performance improvement and risk management outcomes ➤ Maintains historical program data ➤ Obtains input/feedback from key stakeholders	Utilizes tools and processes to plan education and validation programs.
Data Analysis	➤ Organizes and formats data ➤ Identifies trends and patterns ➤ Assesses measurement criteria ➤ Attests to validity and reliability ➤ Distinguishes competency versus performance issues	Synthesizes needs assessment outcomes.
Program Design	➤ Develops programs with written purpose, goals, and objectives ➤ Develops content ➤ Uses a variety of methodology of program delivery ➤ Utilizes current evidence-based references and resources ➤ Develops participant and program outcome measures ➤ Adheres to regulatory and accreditation standards ➤ Demonstrates use of best practices and community standards ➤ Provides accurate record keeping	Uses education theory and data analysis to structure and plan curriculum.

Needs Assessment

Needs assessments are conducted to identify and prioritize learning needs. Assessing *needs* and assessing *interests* are two very different assessments; be clear on what you are assessing. Also, differentiate learning need from system or performance problems and meeting accreditation standards. This assessment process provides a guide for program development. Conducting a needs assessment is an important skill the educator must develop. Development of a good assessment tool is a competency which is learned over time through mentorship by experienced educators or through trial and error (Avillion, 2008).

Needs assessment is a systematic exploration of the practice as it is and the way practice should be. The educator must identify what skills, knowledge, and abilities are needed in comparison to current staff performance. Determining the educational needs of staff in ambulatory care has many facets. One has to take into consideration the organization's culture and goals. The organization's mission, vision, values, and strategic plan provide a framework for what direction the nurse educator should take in assessing needs and planning programs. Knowing what resources the organization is willing to provide, both financial and human, identifies boundaries within which the educator must perform. An effective needs assessment can ensure training dollars are used effectively.

The educator must define the skill, knowledge, and abilities needed by staff to meet job expectations. Information can be collected from various sources. Interviews, questionnaires or surveys, focus groups, input from management, performance evaluations, and tests provide input from the key stakeholders, who are staff and supervisors. Organizational sources include quality improvement audit findings, policy and procedure changes, job descriptions, incident reports, review of community standards, and patient complaints. Patient satisfaction surveys can also provide insight into societal expectations. Healthcare reform has stimulated intense public interest in access to health care, quality, and cost. These expectations are fed by the media, Internet access to information, the litigious atmosphere of the country, our aging population, and reports in the media of medical errors. These factors in the community environment affect public opinion as well as staff's perceptions and expectations (National Nursing Staff Development Organization [NNSDO], 2001).

Planning is imperative for creating a valid needs assessment tool. Determine a focus or goal by answering these three questions:
- What specific problem or problems need to be corrected?
- Will education correct the problem? If so, how?
- Who needs the education?

Identify what you want to find out. Examples could be:
- How can we improve staff performance?
- What are the staff's personal growth needs?
- What are the needs of staff to improve patient care?
- What is the effectiveness of current programs?

Identify your target audience. Rarely is education a one size fits all. Keep it simple. Long surveys tend to lose your audience before they complete the survey. This decreases the usable data you collect (Avillion, 2008).

Word the questions so you get usable answers. Example: you want to know the effectiveness of your online lessons. Asking, "What online lessons do you value most?" may not provide usable data. If you list all of the lessons you want feedback on and have the person rate each lesson on a scale of 1-3 (1 – not helpful, 2 – helpful, 3 – must have, NA – lesson not used by my department), you are more likely to identify lessons that can be removed or that need to be revised.

Ask, "Can the data you plan to collect be managed in the computer?" If so, this is a major time-saver when faced with tabulating multiple data points on multiple surveys (Donner, Levonian, & Slutsky, 2005). There are a number of free online survey tools that can be used such as SurveyMonkey, Zoomerang, and Vista.

Surveys are an effective way to collect data to assess training or educational needs. However, surveys are subjective in nature and staff do not always know what they do not know; therefore, it should not be your only source of information. Develop a process for educational requests to be communicated to the education department (The Staff Educator, Jan. 2009). Risk managers can supply information of errors being reported. The quality improvement department can provide information from their studies that identify knowledge or skill deficits that may be improved by education. Nurse managers or supervisors may provide real-time issues that need addressing. Testing and interviewing of the staff provides a better understanding of staff needs and perspectives.

Focus groups can be facilitated by asking open-ended questions. Working with a small group of 10 or less, staff affords the educator an opportunity to discuss current challenges, analyze potential costs, identify preferred format, and preferred time and place for education delivery. When working with a group, it is important that care be taken not to introduce personal biases. Remember non-verbal communication can influence the group as easily as verbal. Your goal is to gain perspective on the needs of the staff and unit. If the group only tells you what they think you want to hear, you have wasted everyone's time. When receiving information, identify the problem, the barriers, any underlying issues, and how others are contributing to the problem. It is prudent to also know what action has already been taken and its effectiveness (The Staff Educator, May 2008).

Evidenced-based practice is demonstrated through nursing practice indicators related to staffing issues, assessment skills, and patient outcomes. It has become important to develop and implement research in daily practice to solve unsolved questions, offer new solutions to old issues, and work with colleagues to optimize care through integrative practice solutions (Attwood, 2009). Evidenced-based interventions are defined by multidisciplinary care teams of physicians, nurses, pharmacists, radiologists, laboratory staff, dietitians, and others sharing ideas and developing creative ways to improve patient care. The nurse educator must keep a watchful eye on the rapid changes in practice standards as more evidence-based care initiatives are validated.

The National Quality Forum (NQF) has developed voluntary standards for ambulatory care focusing on management of chronic diseases and disease prevention (www.qualityforum.org/nursing/). The educator should review the evidence, understand current work flows, and develop educational initiative to keep staff abreast of new innovations.

Regulatory guidelines provide a professional frame for program planning. The Joint Commission and Accreditation Association for Ambulatory Health Care provide standards which must be met for accreditation of the organization. The standards provide a benchmark for care excellence. These standards are available on the respective organization's Web sites.

Professional nurse organizations such as American Nurses Association, National Nursing Staff Development Organization, and American Academy of Ambulatory Care Nursing provide resources, guidelines, and written professional standards for the educator. These organizations and agencies provide rich resources which the educator may incorporate into educational initiatives.

Educational Needs Assessment:
A Continuous Process

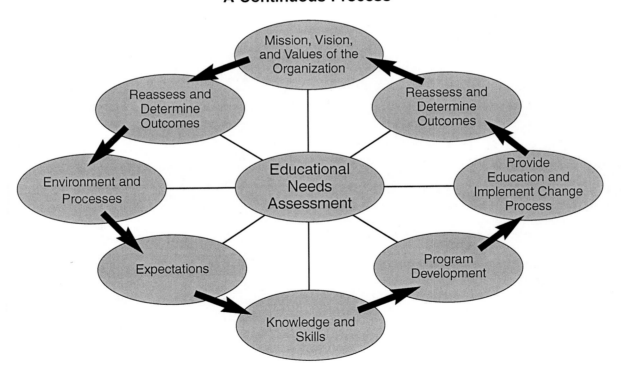

Data Analysis

Once a list of training needs is determined, organize the data into a format that allows the educator to identify priorities and determine the importance of each topic. Know the *what, how,* and *why* of the training need, taking into account the organization's culture. It takes cautious and careful planning to properly assess the priority of educational needs (Rouda & Kusy, 1995). The tendency is to consider any established need for education as an absolute. Few organizations have the resources to address all needs. As the educator, one must make decisions based on resources available for staff education. Do you have the right staff, time, and money? Mandatory training usually gets priority. If time and dollars are still available, the next step is to determine which topic to address. What is the consequence of not providing the training? Compare the benefit of each need. Consider availability of training from outside the organization. The current economic environment places emphasis on quality, cost containment, and efficiency. So, the educator must justify and document the need for education he or she plans to pursue for the staff. Be sure you have distinguished competency verses performance issues. An employee may have the competence but lack a willingness to perform. If attitude is the problem, management will need to fact-find as to the source and take action.

1. Determine what the cost impact is on staffing, materials, and finances. What is the impact of not meeting the need?
2. Determine if there are any legal requirements that are impacted. What is mandated? This could add value to the topic.
3. Determine organizational priorities. Management pressures can change the urgency level given to a topic.
4. Determine the scope of the need. Are there common problems that occur with new employees? Is there new technology being introduced? What competencies have been identified? How many will need to be trained? Is the problem widespread or limited? Is it a small group or the whole facility?
5. Impact on the patient also weighs in on determining the level of priority given a topic. Are there any reports that indicate a patient care problem?

A chart or table may be helpful in identifying priorities by examining the importance and impact of each topic.

List each need and enter impact information. Assign a score for each column. 1 is lowest, 2 is next lowest, etc. The highest number reflects the number of needs identified. An example for 6 identified needs can be seen on p. 126. Each column is rated 1-6, with 6 being most important. Once each column is scored, add the horizontal line for each topic.

The chart helps identify trends and patterns in the data, assisting in the determination of the educational need with the highest priority. When completing the chart, verify the reliability of the information being entered. Take into consideration resources available to the educator. Assess the measurement criteria used to complete the chart. Watch for personal biases. From this chart, one can surmise that the medical assistant program should take priority, followed by the telephone management program.

Summary

The educator planning an educational program begins by assessing the needs of the staff and organization. Using a variety of data collection methods (including historical program data), the educator can develop a plan to meet the educational needs of the organization. Once needs are identified, issues are prioritized and topics that will be address are identified. Validation, input, and feedback from key stakeholders set the stage for the educator to proceed with program development (Staff Educator, Feb. 2009).

Program Design

Once the need for an educational program is identified, objectives, content, and methodology for delivery of the content is determined. In an ambulatory setting, there is the added nuance of the need to make the information available to a variety of staff in a variety of settings. Many ambulatory clinics have multiple sites and/or multiple specialties requiring a diverse and flexible catalog of training events and programs.

Developing Objectives and Learning Activities

Know the purpose for the educational initiative. The purpose may be accomplished by a single goal or it may need several goals. Goal and objective development is a key part of planning for an educational program. A goal is the broad overview of what the student's proficiency will accomplish. For example, a goal for an IV course could be that at the end of the training, the learner would be proficient in starting and maintaining intravenous therapy. An objective is the narrower statement of an observable and measurable behavior. For the IV course, an objective could be that the learner "demonstrates a safe and effective IV start." Objectives are always stated behaviorally; they may reflect knowledge, comprehension, application, analysis, synthesis, or evaluation. Clear measurable objectives not only facilitate content development, but allow the instructor to measure and evaluate the success of the training. If the objectives are not met, they allow the instructor to regroup and improve the course. Objectives must include the expected behavior of the target audience at the completion of the course. They are always verbs and demonstrate a measurable outcome of the class by the participant. Objectives can be broken down into sever-

Example Chart

Need	Impact if Not Met	Legal Impact	Management Interest	Scope of Need	Impact on Patients	Score
Annual Skills Assessment	Could impact accreditation status 4	Required for accreditation 1	High 3	All clinical staff 6	No immediate 1	15
Code Blue Training	Could impact accreditation; may increase risk of legal action 3	Required for accreditation 4	High 4	All clinical staff 4	Poor outcome if emergency response mismanaged 3	18
CPR	Could impact accreditation 5	Required for accreditation 3	Moderate 2	All clinical staff 5	Poor outcome if emergency response mismanaged 2	17
Immunization Training	No immediate 1	CDC provide frequent updates for immunization compliance 2	Moderate 1	New staff. Pedi, IM, & FM nurses 3	Poor outcome if nurse provides incorrect immunization counseling or gives wrong vaccine 5	12
Medical Assistant (MA) Training	Improve patient flow and increase physician productivity 6	Physician delegates to MA; nurse trains, verifies competency and provides supervision; staff need to function within scope of practice 6	High 6	MAs are 30% of clinical staff 2	Medication error if not trained 4	24
Telephone Management	Increased risk from incomplete or inaccurate messaging 2	RNs may triage; LPN/LVNs may use protocols working with physician or RN to take messages 5	High 5	Large volume of calls per day RN and LPN/LVNs answering phones 1	Poor out come or delay of care if call mishandled 6	19

al categories; knowledge, comprehension, application, analysis, synthesis, or evaluation. Each category has many verbs that will provide a measurable statement reflecting the student's assimilation of the information. Below are a few examples of each.

Knowledge	Comprehension	Application
• Define	• Discuss	• Demonstrate
• Record	• Explain	• Practice
• List	• Define	• Illustrate
• Name	• Locate	• Apply
• State	• Recognize	• Employ
Analysis	**Synthesis**	**Evaluation**
• Classify	• Plan	• Rate
• Differentiate	• Create	• Evaluate
• Analyze	• Design	• Assess
• Test	• Summarize	• Compare
• Examine	• Organize	• Select

A lesson plan is a tool that facilitates bringing all of your ideas and strategies into one product. Educators use them very early in the planning stage as they help discern if the time allotted is realistic and the objectives are clear and possible for the allowed length of time.

Choosing and Recruiting Speakers/Presenters

Occasionally speakers will volunteer to do a presentation or contact the educator with an idea for a training program or class. Other speakers may be suggested by staff, physicians, or your peers. Maintain a roster of contacts or people who have spoken in the past. Make a list of excellent speakers and their topics when attending workshops or conferences. Clinical experts may be utilized to present in their areas of expertise. Being an expert does not always correlate with great speaking or teaching ability. It then becomes a role for the educators to mentor and support their trainers in the fine art of public speaking and development of a program. Novice presenters may need help creating content to meet objectives and some training on how to best reach the adult learner.

Know Your Learners

It is important to assess your learners' experiences, as they can have an impact on your program. Ambulatory clinic staffs often come from other venues, nursing homes, hospitals, or home care. It is helpful to find out what each participant already knows in order to teach at a level that is meaningful for them. Each participant may be at a different place in his or her learning development.

Adult learners also need to be engaged and feel a connection with the speakers and the classes. They will quickly lose interest if they do not feel that the information being presented is pertinent to them. You should be able to maintain the audience's interest by interspersing lecture with hands-on practice, demonstrations, and question and answer sessions.

Begin the development of an educational offering by determining your target audience. Who will be the learners in this program? In some settings, there may be a need to produce a program for several types of employees and multiple levels of health care providers. For example, registered nurses only (e.g., IV skills); RNs, LPNs/LVNs, and medical assistants (e.g., charting updates, immunization review); or physicians only (e.g., patient satisfaction, listening well).

Topic	Goals and Objectives	Learning Activity	Time	Evaluation
Peripheral IV Starts **Learners:** RN **Format:** Classroom Six or fewer students	Goal(s): Learner will be able to start an IV on a practice arm. Objectives: At the end of the workshop, the learner will: 1. Demonstrate a successful IV start with a blood flashback on the demo arm. 2. Describe an effective dressing technique for a peripheral IV. 3. Choose an appropriate IV catheter size based on patient and fluid or medication being infused.	Lecture with demonstration. Supplies needed: • Handouts • IV trays • Gloves • Alcohol wipes • IV demo arm • Tubing • Tegaderm, gauze, and tape • Bag of IV fluid Return demonstration. Venipuncture on demo arm; prep and dressing on other student.	40 min. 20 min.	Skill demonstrated; skills checklist completed.

Adults learn best when they understand the importance of what they are learning. When working in a training situation, it is necessary to make the information relevant to the student's work or life. They do well if they feel that the new information will help them or their patients, and they can clearly see that the learning offers them something meaningful.

Adult learners are more responsive after a major event has occurred. Students will often tell you that they need feedback whenever they do something well or when something goes wrong. Think of your first medication error; was your mentor understanding or punitive? A discussion of what the error was as well as the impact on the patient develops critical thinking skills and provides a great lesson on counseling a peer (Mergel, 1998).

Class Format

It is important to address the differences in learning styles and preferences with all learners in all of these groups. There are many ways to present material, and these choices are also to be considered early in the planning. The decision to develop a class may be to have a traditional classroom program, lecture and discussion, offer one-on-one training with hands on practice, or e-learning with a test and skills check-off. This could be a recurring class or a one-time offering. You need to know if this class is mandatory or optional, and whether continuing education for nurses, physicians, or other credit will be provided. All of these questions need to be answered in the early stages of program planning.

Other considerations for the class may be to determine if it is part of a general core competency program, a continuing part of orientation, or a one-time offering.

Once you have determined your audience, you must develop a timeline. The goals and objectives for the topic will guide the development of the presentation. Estimate how much time will be needed to plan. As a rule of thumb, it may take up to 4 hours to plan one hour of content.

To develop a one or two day seminar with multiple speakers, it may be helpful to use a program planning spreadsheet that reminds you of all of the tasks to perform with set deadlines and responsibility assigned. This is a process that could take six or more months of planning. A venue must be found. Decide how large an audience you will need to target, and whether or not meals will be provided. At the same time, a tentative agenda is developed, which drives your decision about which speakers should be contacted. Once speakers are set, work with them to meet your objectives. If requesting nursing contact hours, the appropriate application is completed. Grant application may also be needed. Allow time to make handouts or a syllabus. This could easily take several months. On the other hand, a new one-hour class may take a month or less of program planning.

One way to track planning progress is using a table with the timeline for each step and the status. For example:

Program Description	Tasks	Person Responsible	Target Date	Complete
Peripheral IV Training: A two-hour course and lab to sign off on peripheral IV insertion, dressing, and removal.	• Set dates and reserve classroom	Instructor	• Jan. 15, 2011	Rm. 1 reserved for every Friday in March, 1-3 pm
	• Develop outline for module		• Feb. 3, 2011	•
	• Order supplies for class		• Feb 1, 2011	•
	• Finalize handouts and PowerPoint presentation		• Feb 12, 2011	•

Method of Delivery

In creating a training plan, determine the training methodology that works best for the delivery of the topic. What teaching format provides the best learning experience for the student to meet the objectives? Sound objectives will drive methodology as well. For example, an objective to demonstrate the correct placement of a peripheral IV might define the need to have discussion on IV placement principles, demonstration with learner practice, and return demonstration.

Consider classroom presentation, online self-directed materials and testing, small group interactive workshop, role plays, skills lab demonstration and practice, or a combination. With limited resources, remember that classroom-based programs may not be appropriate for all topics or situations. A topic or need may be met by providing clear-cut guidelines in a self-directed handout. It is important to determine the most appropriate teaching methodology to engage participants in learning and mastering the required skill or knowledge. As educational needs are addressed, a continuation of assessment and evaluation must be maintained.

Common Methodology Used to Deliver Education

Methodology	Pros	Cons
Lecture – Classroom Presentation	Most efficient.	Passive interaction.
Written or Online Self-Directed Materials	Scheduling flexibility. Learner can proceed at his/her own pace.	No Q&A time. May need computer access.
Video/DVD	Realistic/independent use. Can enhance classroom presentations.	Passive. Requires equipment.
Internet	Wide variety of options on topics. Self-paced.	Material may not be applicable. Need computer access.
Visual Aids	PowerPoint presentation easy to use. Enhances lectures.	Need computer access. May need training on PowerPoint software.
Case Studies	Realistic. Promotes critical thinking.	Time-consuming. Takes a lot of planning. Needs experienced instructor.
Demonstrations	Communicates performance expectations. Can stress correct execution of difficult aspects.	Best for small groups. Need supplies. Takes time.

Source: NNSDO, 2001.

References/Resources

These are key to program development. A literature search on the Internet provides access to the latest research and best practices. Written materials such as journals, position statements, and white papers from related professional organizations are rich sources of information. AAACN provides a voice for ambulatory care nursing. National Nursing Staff Development Organization (NNSDO) provides a wide variety of tools for the educator to improve his or her skills as an instructor. Don't forget to utilize expert staff (nurse practitioners, clinical nurse specialists, and physicians) as resources when creating programs.

Participant and Program Outcome Measures

Create a written evaluation tool, verify behavioral changes through clinical behavior observation, or team with the Quality Improvement department to assess documentation improvements in chart audits. Program evaluation is discussed in detail in a later chapter of this book.

Educational Program

This must include regulatory and accreditation standards. The Joint Commission and AAACN provide standards for accreditation of ambulatory care organizations; ANCC provides guidelines for Continuing Nurse Education; HIPAA, Occupational Safety and Health Administration (OSHA), and Centers for Medicare & Medicaid Services (CMS) provide governmental guidelines for practice; National Committee for Quality Assurance (NCQA) defines quality standards.

Record-Keeping

Tracking who has received education or training and what was taught guides the educator in the direction programs should go next. Review of evaluations helps improve ongoing programs and create new ones. Future needs assessments can be drawn from training records. Maintaining accurate records also helps the organization meet accreditation standards and provides proof of compliance during surveys.

References

Attwood, C.A. (2009). Using the evidence to develop ambulatory-specific indicators. *ViewPoint, 31*(1), 12-13.

Avillion, A. (2008). *A practical guide to staff development: Evidence-based tools and techniques for effective education.* Marblehead, MA: HCPro, Inc.

Donner, C.L., Levonian, C., & Slutsky, P. (2005). Move to the head of the class: Developing staff nurses as teachers. *Journal for Nurses in Staff Development, 21*(6), 277-283.

Huang, J. (2006). Inquiry on the essences of learning organization. *Journal of Adult Higher Education, 6.*

Mergel, B. (1998). *Instruction design and learning theory.* Retrieved from http://www.usask.ca/education/coursework/802paper/merel/brenda.htm

Mitchell, M.L., & Courtney, M. (2005). Improving transfer from the intensive care unit: The development, implementation and evaluation of a brochure based on Knowles' Adult Learning Theory. *International Journal of Nurse Practice, 11*(6), 257-268.

National Nursing Staff Development Organization (NNSDO). (2001). *Getting started in clinical and nursing development* (2nd ed.). Pensacola, FL: Author.

Rouda, R.H., & Kusy, M.E. Jr. (1995). *Needs assessment: The first step.* Retrieved from http://www.work911.com/pages/Training/Training_Needs_Assessment/

Staff Educator, The. (May 2008). *Competency corner.* Vol. 4, No. 5. Marblehead, MA: HCPro, Inc.

Staff Educator, The. (Jan. 2009). *Competency corner.* Vol. 5, No. 1. Marblehead, MA: HCPro, Inc.

Staff Educator, The. (Feb. 2009). *Competency corner.* Vol. 5, No. 2. Marblehead, PA: HCPro, Inc.

Chapter 8

The Learning Environment and Program Development

Carol Brautigam, MSN, RN

The learning environment incorporates the educator, the program content, the participants, and the physical setting. It is the educator's competency that stimulates learners to be willing to change their behavior and incorporate new knowledge and skills into their health care practice.

Introduction

Staff development specialists in ambulatory care are called upon to provide timely education to meet the needs of a quickly changing health care delivery system which must provide quality outcomes to patients. Development of education programs requires attention to organization goals and objectives, determination of key stake holders, the participant mix, and the type of information to be disseminated. This section will summarize information that can be incorporated into program content and delivery.

Student success is the delivery of the right information to the right person, in the right way, and at the right time. Education success is the effectiveness of the education on meeting desired goals or objectives. The Program Evaluation section (Chapter 9) will address both the effectiveness of the education on individual learning and on the organization goals.

Key Action Tips:

Involve the student/participant by:
- Application of adult learning principles
- Use of creative and diverse teaching strategies and modalities
- Addressing learning styles
- Providing for multicultural and multigenerational participants
- Determining audience level and comprehension
- Managing resistant participants
- Responding to educational needs with flexibility and spontaneity

Example

New employee orientation at Community Medical Clinic provides the organization mission, history, OSHA and HIPAA requirements, customer service, computer training, and benefits to newly hired employees. The orientation program extends over two days and is offered twice a month. All employees attend this program. Employees vary in age from 18 to 60 and over. There are significant employees of Asian and Hispanic background. Attendance may vary over the year from 10 to 30 persons per class. To meet organization cost containment goals, the Staff Development Department has been asked to reduce the length of the classroom program to one day twice a month. The education specialists must refine this program to meet organizational and individual participant needs.

Delivery of the right information to the right person, in the right way, at the right time is a requirement of staff development educators.

Subtopic	Elements	Competency Statement
Learning Environment – Establishes an Atmosphere That Facilitates Student Success	➤ Adult learning principles ➤ Creative and diverse teaching strategies ➤ Communication styles ➤ Audience level and comprehension ➤ Learning styles ➤ Multicultural and multigenerational considerations ➤ Flexibility and spontaneity ➤ Strategies for resistant participants ➤ Informatics ➤ Classroom location and set-up	Employs and facilitates techniques that hold student interest and attention.

ADULT LEARNING PRINCIPLES

There are four well-established characteristics of adult learning. The goal of utilizing adult learning principles is to improve staff performance, resulting in an increase in the quality of health care provided to patients. The effectiveness of the adult learning principals depends upon their application to the learning strategies employed in the presentation (Avillion, 2005, pp. 41-48).

1. Adults are self-directed learners
   - Advertise the purpose of the education
   - Offer the program at times and in a way that is as convenient as possible
   - Provide clear learning objectives
   - Share the impact of their learning on patient care (e.g., percent improvement in an area)
2. Adults bring life experience to the learning situation
   - Encourage sharing of relevant experience
   - Give credit to staff who provided experiences for distance learning
   - Treat experiences with respect
3. Adults focus on knowledge and skills needed to perform their job or improve their own life
   - Provide opportunities for mandatory education to be challenged with an exam or competency skill check for those whose role frequently utilizes specific skill sets
4. Adults respond to both internal and external motivators
   - Intrinsic motivators include increased self-esteem, job satisfaction, and ability to manage stress
   - Extrinsic motivators include promotions, salary increases, improved job opportunities, and better working conditions
   - Incorporate motivators into the education

CREATIVE AND DIVERSE TEACHING STRATEGIES

There is need to address the ever-changing nursing issues, technology, organizational and professional values, license and certification requirements, department processes, and legal compliance with a variety of learner-effective and cost-effective methods. Ways that nurses learn include: ask for help, watch someone else do it, look it up (printed or online), journal reading, educated guess, and continuing education. Teaching strategies and modalities can address each of these learning methods.

E-Learning/Distance Learning

Distance learning was originally paper- and pencil-based. While this format is sometimes used, more and more frequently distance education is being provided by e-learning. Distance learning has expanded the possibilities for providing timely education to multiple staff members in a cost-effective manner. It has added a new dimension to the learning environment. E-learning/distance learning incorporates audio conferences, video conferences, and computer-based learning. Computer-based learning ranges from DVD or video, which provide individual learning, to interactive Webinars. Distance learning is an $11 billion a year industry (Mangold, 2007, pp. 21-23).

E-learning advantages:
- Interactive or individual learning opportunities
- Endless opportunity to offer the course or program
- Easy to build and use for quick response to new requests or requirements

E-learning requirements:
- Software platform with license agreement
- Availability of appropriate computer hardware
- Keep responses to simple point and click

E-learning is usually thought of as computer-based, but also includes:
- Audio conference
- Transfer of information from traditional lecture to CD format with and without audio (individual learning)
- Video conference
- Webinar
- Videos and DVDs

Simulation and Skill Demonstration

Simulation varies from multiple types of equipment set-ups, to use of traditional models and manikins, to electronically-controlled manikins. The American Heart Association course scenarios are a common example of collaborative learning. Equipment education is often provided online and is an example of individual learning by simulation. No matter how simple or complex the equipment or skill being demonstrated, debriefing and feedback following the demonstration are key to having the greatest educational impact from the simulation/demonstration.

Advantages of simulation:
- Allows individual and collaborative learning
- Provides multiple opportunities to improve skill sets
- Provides practice with high-risk patient situations in a safe environment
- Offers role-playing opportunities for multiple health care team members, patients, and family
- Traditional Mock Code scenarios are an example of collaborative learning

- Computer-controlled manikins have expanded the patient situations presented to staff
- Incorporates role-playing, offering multiple roles for group practice (patient, nurse, physician, family, and other health care team members)
- Video taped for analysis by participants and others
- Allows practice and re-practice for high-risk situations
- Summary debriefing provides feedback to the participants

Requirements of electronic simulation:
- Computer hardware and appropriate manikins/models
- Development of scenarios
- Storage space
- Adequate space for implementation of scenarios and debriefing
- Video recording equipment for scenario analysis
- Transport capability to reach multiple sites

Traditional Lecture/Class

Centuries of lecture as the primary mode for education have led many to expect and enjoy it. Others dislike it. Varying the communication style can help involve more of the participants in the learning process. Lecture can be varied and made interactive by incorporating dialogue, discussion, small group work, and role-playing. Dialogue invites the learner to question the facts of the information presented and to analyze cause and effect of conflicts or issues raised by new information. Not all generations or cultures are comfortable expressing issues or problems for others to solve. There may also be discomfort with the subject matter.

Enhancement of the lecture:
- PowerPoint presentations
- Handouts
- Incorporates interaction with educator and participants through discussion, role-playing, and case presentations (Avillion, 2005, pp. 71-75)
- Requires educator to be focused on outcomes, be enthusiastic about the topic, and be entertaining, all in balance

Small group (traditional in-service education):
- Allows staff discussion and input
- Requires skilled facilitation to maintain focus and draw out members who are non-participating

One-on-one instruction and printed self-learning modules are also considered traditional modes of education.

COMMUNICATION STYLES
Dialogue as a Style Apart From Lecture

Advantages: Invites learner to question the facts of the information presented, to analyze cause and effect of conflicts or issues new information raises, and redefines understanding of issues that reflect the learner's reality.

Limitations: Not all are comfortable expressing issues or problems for others to solve; discomfort with self-directed learning; poor communicators; discomfort with subject matter.

Promote dialogue in advertising courses by mentioning problem-solving teaching, small group work, Q & A interviewing, role-playing, and case study work.

LEARNING STYLES

Auditory, visual, and *kinesthetic* (psychomotor) are the learning styles that have been identified for many years. The information on learning styles must be incorporated into the education planning for it to be of value. Further, the educator must recognize his or her own learning style and provide for the other styles as well (Avillion, 2005, pp. 91-95).
1. Expect to be teacher/faculty-led. The result of centuries of practice. Need orientation to newer hands-on styles of teaching.
2. Take on own project to solve a problem or apply new information right away. May view online courses as training versus education. Pragmatic individuals.
3. Motivation comes from a need to fulfill a professional gap or direction from superiors.
4. Rely on friends or colleagues who are professional experts when seeking advice on learning or starting a new educational effort. This is done in place of doing one's own research on the topic as it applies to one's personal preferences. This may result in disappointment because one's own preferences were not built into the decision process.
5. Want to contribute to the discussion and have those contributions acknowledged. Courses will be more successful if there is a way for the student to take a leadership role (discussion leader or handout contributor).

Auditory Learners (Avillion, 2005, pp. 91-95)
Learn by hearing and responding to auditory directions
Characteristics of auditory learners:
- Talk to themselves, hum when bored
- Read aloud to learn
- Tone of their voice reveals their emotions
- Want to talk through problems or procedures

Best learning situations:
- Audio conferences
- Audio tapes
- Discussions
- Lecture format

Handouts and visual aides are less important to them.

Visual Learners
Predominant learning style for adults
Characteristics of visual learners:
- Sit where they can see
- Detailed, copious notes
- Like use of imagery in discussion and verbal presentation
- May close eyes to visualize what learning
- Facial affect reveals their emotions
- Like colorful, illustrated, easy to read handouts

Kinesthetic Learners (Psychomotor/Hands-on)
Learn by physical involvement
Characteristics of kinesthetic learners:
- Speak with their hands, display emotions with body language
- Require frequent breaks
- Skill demonstration works well for them
- Tone of voice may reflect their emotion

It is important that the educator recognize his/her own learning style and provide for other styles as well.

AUDIENCE LEVEL AND COMPREHENSION
(Evaluation of individual understanding versus program outcome)

Determine Audience Level
- Background knowledge, reading level, learning styles, professional roles, ESL participants

Clinical and Orientation Considerations
(Burns, Beauchesne, Ryan-Krause, & Sawin, 2006)
- Participation, repetition, reinforcement enhance learning
- Variety in learning activities increases interest
- Readiness to learn (from interest) enhances retention
- Immediate use of information and skills enhances retention
- Determine level of ability (high or low level of experience/novice to expert)
- Structured approach versus sink or swim
- Modeling
- Observation
- Case presentation
- Direct questioning

Determine Audience Comprehension

MULTICULTURAL AND MULTIGENERATIONAL CONSIDERATIONS
U.S.A. Generations

Cultural and generational sensitivity requires knowledge of various cultures and generations so there is awareness of the potential behaviors and expectations of persons from different cultures and generations (Avillion, 2005, pp. 104, 110).

When providing cultural sensitive training, include the cultural characteristics of the most frequently encountered cultures.

When delivering presentations, pay attention to the communication behavior of the participants. Knowing some of the commonly encountered behaviors will enable you to properly respond to the participants of varying cultures (Avillion, 2005, pp. 107-109).
- Head of household/family
- Role of women
- Role of elderly
- Role of children
- Importance of children
- Gender value of children
- Role of extended family
- Family structure
- Decision-maker for health care
- Communication behavior (eye contact, gestures, body language, voice, spokesperson)
- Sexuality (gender roles, sexual orientation, circumcision, menstruation, birth control, birth process)
- Pain (perception [punishment]), expression, measures to relieve pain)
- Diet and nutrition (role of religion)
- Religion (influence on illness/injury perception, treatment issues)
- Health practices (home remedies, cultural remedies, trust in eastern or western medicine, end-of-life issues)
- Work ethic (gender issues, financial need, respect of specific occupations)
www.ggalanti.com/articles.html

Traditional
1900-1945   75 million   (Futch, 2003)
- Culture: saving, avoid waste, do without or with little
- Major events: WWI, Depression, WWII, Korean War, Bay of Pigs

- Major figures: FDR, Joe DiMaggio, Joe Louis, Dr. Spock, Duke Ellington, Ella Fitzgerald, John Wayne, Betty Crocker
- Values: Loyalty, patriotism, hard work, work together

Baby Boomers
1946-1964   80 million   (Mangold, 2007)
- Culture: Prosperous culture with nuclear family intact
- Major events: TV, man on the moon, Kennedy assassinated, Vietnam War, Civil Rights Act, Watergate, Chappaquiddick, Kent State
- Major figures: Martin Luther King, Jr., Richard Nixon, JFK, Eldridge Cleaver, Gloria Steinem, Kingston Trio, Elvis Presley, Beatles, Janis Joplin
- Values: "workaholic," service oriented, optimistic, desire personal gratification
- Learning environment was traditional lecture, want a comfortable learning environment, desire positive feedback
- Learning preference is process-oriented (what and how before the why)

Generation X
1965-1980   46 million   (Futch, 2003)
- Culture: Tripled divorce rate, single-parent homes, latch key kids, failed institutions and heroes
- Major events: cable TV, microwaves, cell phones, computer, Palm Pilots®
- Major figures: Bill Gates, Bill Clinton, Monica Lewinsky, Ayatollah Khomeini, Clarence Thomas, Beavis and Butt-Head, Dilbert, Madonna, Michael Jordon
- Values: self-command

Millennial (Generation Y)
1981-1999/2001   76 million   (Avillion, 2005; Futch, 2003; Mangold, 2007)
- Culture: 30% raised in single-parent families, 34% of ethnic minority, raised to be very busy (school, multiple outside activities)
- Major events: technological boom, chat rooms, Monica Lewinsky scandal, Oklahoma City Bombing and 9-11, economic downturn
- Major figures: Prince William, Chelsea Clinton, Britney Spears, Mark McGuire, Sammy Sosa, Venus and Serena Williams
- Values: technology is required, public safety, saving money, civic-minded, value diversity, reading, collaboration
- Learning preference is digitally- and interactively-oriented, doing rather than knowing, trial and error versus reading a manual, little

tolerance for delays, need to stay connected (communication multitasking of surfing the Internet, talking on cell phone, and listening to music at the same time)
- Simulation preferred because it is fun, interactive, provides team experience, offers immediate feedback

Cuspers span each generation and are experts at mediating, translating, and mentoring the spanned generations (Futch, 2003):
- Traditionalists/Baby Boomer (1940-1945)
- Baby Boomer/Generation X (1960-1965)
- Generation X/Millennial (1975-1980)

"Generations" have shared the same set of life experiences in society at about the same point in their development (Mangold, 2007).

FLEXIBILITY AND SPONTANEITY
- The ability to adapt content to the knowledge base, learning styles, generations, and cultural variables present in a live class.
- Provide content in more than one venue (classroom, department in-service) and in more than one modality (ground/online classes)

STRATEGIES FOR RESISTANT PARTICIPANTS
Participants who are seen as resistive to the education may be frustrated, bored, ill, and dissatisfied. For mandatory education and competence demonstration, they may fear failure. Resistant participants interrupt a positive learning environment. The goal is to defuse them (Burns et al., 2006).

Methods to reduce resistant participants:
- Provide the purpose of the learning activity
- Determine if the learning activity is a response to a learning need or a systems flaw
- Provide for various learning styles, cultural and generational characteristics
- Design learning for maximum effectiveness to minimize negative consequences of failure (probation, termination)
- Educator is respected for both their education and experience (qualified)
- Apply new knowledge and skills to the work setting
- Provide supportive physical and emotional learning environments
- The educator is enthusiastic about what is being taught

Hostile participants:
- Provide a break in the class and speak privately with the participant(s)
- Make sure the participant can effectively respond to the type of education offered (computer skills)
- Participant may fear failure and its consequences

Violent participants:
- Sit and ask them to sit
- Be sure you have access to the exit of the room (ask the participant to leave or leave yourself)
- Avoid threatening gestures
- Use a calm, measured voice
- Realize the anger is probably displaced
- Listen actively
- Know how to get help quickly; have a colleague present with you
- Report all incidents of violence (verbal or physical) (Avillion, 2005, pp. 121-129)

INFORMATICS

Distance learning or e-learning has revolutionized staff education, allowing for cost-effective, convenient, and just in time learning. It has several requirements for both the development of the education product and its use (Avillion, 2005, pp. 73-75).

CLASSROOM LOCATION AND SET-UP

Florence Nightingale emphasized the importance of lighting in patient care: adequate light, not too bright, the caregiver not back-lighted, the healing and positive effect of light. It is also true for classroom teaching. Often there are not many choices in the rooms assigned for education. There may not be daylight, or the daylight may be glaring. Make use of soft lights and adjust blinds to avoid glare. Configure tables and chairs for the size of the group – modify seating for a small group set-up or for a large one. The educator does not always need to be standing at the front. Being seated near the participants of a small group adds intimacy to the group and increases sharing and dialogue. Provide information on refreshment and restroom facilities when this is not in the participant's office setting.

E-learning requires computer access in a quiet area, not the nursing desk during work hours. Lighting is particularly important to avoid screen glare. Ergonomic chair and computer height need to be accounted for. If there is testing involved, what are the regulations regarding leaving the computer?

Simulation with electronically-controlled manikins may require extensive set-up and adequate space for the simulation. When transportation of this heavy equipment is needed to provide for learning, perhaps miles from the storage site, plan for physical assistance with the moving of the equipment, adequate travel, and set-up time.

References

Avillion, A.E. (2005). *Nurse educator manual.* Marblehead, MA: HCPro, Inc.

Burns, C., Beauchesne, M., Ryan-Krause, P., & Sawin K. (2006). Mastering the preceptor role: Challenges of clinical teaching. *Journal of Pediatric Health Care, 20*(3), 172-183.

Futch, C. (2003). Generations and community: Who are we? *ViewPoint, 25*(5), 5-7.

Mangold, K. (2007). Educating a new generation teaching baby boomer faculty about millennial students. *Nurse Educator, 32*(1), 21-23.

Additional Readings

Jaobson, J. (2007, August 24). *Communication in business and in the work place.* Retrieved from http://EzineArticles.com

Mohatta, C.D. (2007, November 17). *How are your communication skills?* Retrieved from http://EzineArticles.com

NAS Recruitment Communications. (2007). *Recruiting and managing the generations* [White paper]. Cleveland, OH.

Outten, D. (2008, February 8). *Is there a need for soft skills and effective communication in the workplace?* Retrieved from http://EzineArticles.com

Robert Wood Johnson Foundation (RWJF). (2009). *Profile: Amy Barton, QSEN Collaborative Member.* Retrieved from http://www.rwjf.org/pr/product.jsp?id=40213

Chapter 9

Program Evaluation

Kathy Kesner, MS, RN, CNS

Program evaluation is the systematic collection of information about the activities, characteristics, and outcomes of programs to make judgments about the program, improve program effectiveness, and/or inform decisions about future program development (CDC, 2008). Consider it the blueprint of where you are going and how you plan to get there.

Introduction

Evaluation has always been a part of nursing education. In recent years, nurse educators have been asked to expand their scope of program evaluation to ensure that information gained by the participants is comprehensive, useful, and beneficial to both participants and the organization (Burke, 2008). Effective program evaluation allows staff educators to detect a program's effects in a timely manner, which affords the opportunity to be flexible with the teaching strategies to meet the participants' needs. The goals and purpose of an educational program evaluation are to:

- Identify program participants
- Measure the achievement of identified outcomes
- Improve a program's ability to meet the needs of the staff
- Demonstrate effectiveness/value of the program to all stakeholders

Program evaluation is an important practice, and should be integrated into any educational program using realistic, ongoing strategies that involve all stakeholders. How a program will be evaluated should be decided while the program is being developed. Four steps have been identified by Kak, Burkhalter, and Cooper (2001) to ensure that the evaluation portion of a program is effective:

- Utility: Did you learn what you wanted to from the evaluation?
- Feasibility: Is the evaluation practical to carry out?
- Propriety: Is your evaluation method ethical?
- Accuracy: Does your evaluation of the program reflect reality?

Identifying up front what you want to evaluate about the program and how you will do the evaluation is crucial to a program's success.

Key Action Tips

- Establish the goals of the staff education department/program.
- Identify the organization's strategic goals.
- Name key stakeholders and engage them in the process.
- List the goals of the educational offering; define outcomes in measurable terms.
- Focus the evaluation. What aspects of the program do you want to evaluate?
- Share lessons learned with all stakeholders.

Example

The Community Medical Clinic orientation program was reduced to one day. The organization mission, history, and benefits were provided in traditional lecture format. The computer training incorporated delivery of the OSHA, HIPAA, and customer service material in a Web-based format. Evaluation of the new program was planned for assessment at six months and 12 months. Comparisons will be made between the old programs delivered in 2009 to the revised program delivered in 2010. The measures will include educator development time, presentation time, pre-test and post-test results for the content, and feedback from the participants and department managers.

Subtopic	Elements	Competency Statement
Program Evaluation	➤ Purpose, goals, and objectives achievement ➤ Staff competence levels and improvement progression ➤ Operational integration of program content by participants ➤ Staff satisfaction ➤ Stakeholder satisfaction ➤ Direct and indirect correlation of program outcomes to organization's strategic goals ➤ Planning and prioritization of future education programs and teaching strategies	Uses varied feedback and outcomes to appraise program effectiveness.

Purpose, Goals, and Objectives Achievement

When planning staff education, care should be taken to place the horse before the cart. That is, define not only where you are going, but also why and how. The process of developing an educational program should include:

I. Needs assessment of all stakeholders
II. Planning the program to include indentifying the goals. When setting the goals and objectives for the educational program, they should be made specific, measurable, achievable (e.g., do not set a goal that all participants achieve 100% on a knowledge test), relevant, and time-bound.
III. Implementation and ongoing assessment
IV. Evaluation to demonstrate achievement of program goals and evaluate the value of the program to the organization (Clifford, Goldschmidt, & O'Connor, 2007; Hamer, 2008) identified 4 levels for evaluating educational programs:
- How well participants like the program (staff satisfaction)
- Whether or not learning occurred during the program (staff competence/progression)
- Whether or not the program changed behavior (operational integration)
- Whether or not the cost of the program was justified (goals and objectives were met)

Staff Competence Levels and Improvement Progression

Competence assessment is performance evaluation based on expectations set up front. However, confusion continues to exist around the words *competence* and *competency*. Donna Wright defines competence as "the application of knowledge, skills, and behaviors that are needed to fulfill organizational, departmental and work setting requirements" (Wright, 2005, p. 8). Once *competence* is defined for a program, then the level of competence for each set of skills or knowledge must be pre-determined. (Does a score of 90% equate to competence, or do they need to achieve 100%?)

If an employee is not meeting the defined expectation, the educator must determine the reason. One acronym to use is "APES," that is, is it an Attitude, Process, Educational, or Systems problem? Education is only one piece. Having all stakeholders involved in the program from the beginning allows the organization to become aware that not all performance issues are related to education.

Consequences for not meeting the predetermined expectation must be made clear up front. For example, a nurse who does not meet the expectations for post-program competency with peripheral IV starts would not be allowed to start a peripheral IV on a patient until expectations are met. Stakeholder (staff, management, and administration) buy-in for the pre-determined expectations and the consequences of not meeting expectations is crucial.

Operational Integration of Program Content by Participants

One challenge has been that competency does not always lead to effective performance. Competency is often viewed as initial skill and knowledge (skill check-off, test), while performance is viewed as skill in an ongoing, real practice setting. Evaluation of learning must occur to see if knowledge was transferred from the learning setting to the clinical setting (Clifford et al., 2007).

There are steps to take to increase the chance that new knowledge or skills will be applied to practice. Foremost, deliver material in a manner that staff would want to change their practice and feel confident about doing so. Essential to this achievement is using knowledge transfer techniques, such as collaborative teaching and repetitive practice (Hamer, 2008). In addition, there are other factors to consider which affect participant's integration of content (Higgs & Edwards, 1999):

- *Personal factors:* frame of reference, previous knowledge and skills, personal goals, professional characteristics, motivation (increased when participants see an opportunity to demonstrate mastery versus an occasion to be evaluated) and expectations for success
- *Organization, local, and national culture:* culture of safety promotes operationalizing of patient safety skills and knowledge
- *System and process issues:* support, allowing enough time for staff to learn and adjust to changes

Taking these factors into account when planning an educational program will increase the chance that staff will incorporate the knowledge into practice, which is, after all, the primary goal of staff education.

Staff Satisfaction

The challenge in developing competency programs is to make them pertinent to practice, engage the participants, and change practice utilizing the latest standards of care (Sen & Tesoro, 2007). To accomplish this, the programs must be flexible and accommodating to differing learning styles, varying generations, and multiple shifts and days worked. Staff should be identified as key stakeholders at the beginning phases of program development. This allows for their input, thus increasing their ownership of the program. In addition, staff as stakeholders can identify how to make the program pertinent, as well as engaging.

A key part of evaluation of staff satisfaction is to simply ask participants: did they enjoy the program, did they find it beneficial, and will they be able to apply the information to their practice. There are many methods of presenting education to meet participant needs: simulation, mock situation, online learning, self-learning modules, presentation, case studies, and even mock trials. Matching the goals and objectives to the best method of teaching will increase staff satisfaction, and increase the likelihood of meeting the program's goals and objectives. Whenever possible, it is beneficial to teach a skill in more than one way: offer a lecture/presentation and an online learning module, and allow participants to choose the method that best suits them.

Stakeholder Satisfaction

A stakeholder is defined as "anyone with an interest in the outcome of the event" (Burke, 2008, p. 228). Stakeholders are administrators, managers, and staff. They should be part of the program planning from the beginning, starting with the needs assessment. Often, nurse educators simply ask staff what their educational needs are. This seems easier and quicker, but does staff really know everything that they need to learn for their practice? Many times staff believes that their strengths are greatest in the area where they are most familiar. Burke (2008) identified that staff become complacent about these familiar tasks, but that often these tasks had the most potential for improvement and thus had a greater impact on quality of care.

Finally, involving all of the stakeholders has the positive outcome that stakeholders feel more ownership and connection when they are involved in identifying needs and planning the educational program (Burke, 2008). This "buy-in" can increase participant stakeholder's integration of the knowledge into practice, and administrator/manager stakeholders' accountability to hold staff to performance standards.

Direct and Indirect Correlation of Program Outcomes to Organization's Strategic Goals

Providing cost-effective education that meets the organization goals is often the expectation of nurse educators.

To do so, the educator must collaborate with the organization's leaders, taking the following steps:

- The mission of staff education is made clear.
- The organization's strategic goals are understood.
- Stakeholders from administration, management, and staff are identified.
- Stakeholders are involved in the entire process from needs identification to evaluation.

The organization's strategic goals can derive from healthcare reform, organizational performance, liability and ethics issues, risk management, certification (Magnet, nurse-sensitive indicators), and planning for new services. Staff education must align with the identified goals, to ensure stakeholder support as well as to assist the organization to be successful toward meeting its goals.

Planning and Prioritization of Future Education Programs and Teaching Strategies

Identification of staff educational needs should be done in a proactive manner (Burke, 2008). To accomplish this, the goals of nursing education must be made clear; stakeholders need to be identified, and processes must be in place to assess, plan, and implement educational programs. Steps should be taken to identify blind or undiscovered needs (Burke, 2008). This can be accomplished in part by looking at:

- Organizational mission and goals
- Healthcare legislation and policies
- Performance assessments
- Quality improvement data
- Customer feedback
- Low-volume, high-risk, problem-prone skills
- Input from all stakeholders

Identifying undiscovered needs and planning for future needs allows the nurse educator to follow the stages of program development, thus increasing the chances of success. It is important to remember that "the ultimate outcome is to correctly identify true educational needs in order to provide learning opportunities that result in quality staff performance and improved patient outcomes" (Burke, 2008, p. 230).

References

Burke, G. (2008). Forecasting instead of reacting to educational needs. *Journal for Nurses in Staff Development, 24*(5).

Centers for Disease Control and Prevention (CDC). (2008). *Vaccines and immunizations: Immunization program evaluation.* Retrieved from http://www.cdc.gov/vaccines/programs/progeval/default.htm

Clifford, P., Goldschmidt, K., & O'Connor, T. (2007). Staff nurses writing for their peers: Development of self-learning modules. *Journal for Nurses in Staff Development, 23*(6), 283-288.

Hamer, B. (2008). A capacity-building model for implementing a nursing best practice. *Journal for Nurses in Staff Development, 24*(1).

Higgs, J., & Edwards, H. (Eds). (1999). *Educating beginning practitioners.* Boston: Butterworth-Heinemann.

Kak, N., Burkhalter, B., & Cooper, M. (2001). *Measuring the competence of healthcare providers.* Operation Research Issue Paper 2(1). Bethesda, MD: U.S. Agency for International Development (USAID) – Quality Assurance Project.

Sen, M., & Tesoro, M. (2007). A mock trial approach: Nursing competency program. *Journal for Nurses in Staff Development, 23*(6).

Wright, D. (2005). *The ultimate guide to competency assessment in health care* (3rd ed.). Minneapolis, MN: Creative Healthcare Management, Inc.

Chapter 10

Professional Self-Development

Carol Ann Attwood, MLS, AHIP, MPH, RN, C

According to Wright (2005), competency assessment is a dynamic, fluid, and ongoing process. This method is always changing as a response to the environment reflecting the current direction and demands of the organization. For the nurse educator to remain competent, the self-assessment is one method of verifying competency. "Self-assessment is a valid form of competency assessment when applied to the appropriate competencies" (Wright, 2005, p. 106). The nurse educator maintains currency and competency in nursing professional development practice.

Key Action Tips

- Professional nurse organization membership provides support and resources to the educator for self-development and maintaining competency.
- Knowledgeable use of online resources allows the educator to recognize best practices.
- Use of current reference materials from research, journals, and reputable online resources support the educator in creating educational programs.

Example

The staff development nurse educator must be involved in continuing education and personal growth activities to maintain his or her competence as an educator.

Subtopic	Performance Outcome	Competency Statement
Professional Knowledge	➤ Conducts ongoing self-assessment and goal development ➤ Holds membership and actively participates in local and national organizations ➤ Serves as a mentor ➤ Conducts, promotes, and integrates research into practice ➤ Subscribes to professional journals ➤ Leads a journal club ➤ Publishes in professional journals ➤ Develops Web-based training ➤ Participates in professional meetings (officer, chairperson, speaker, poster presenter, etc.) ➤ Engages in clinical practice ➤ Continuing education ➤ Secures state and national certification ➤ Obtains undergrad, graduate, post-graduate, doctorate degree	Conducts professional self-development. Participates in ongoing activities to sustain educator competence.

Conducts Professional Self-Development

Definition:

The professional nursing staff educator participates in ongoing activities to maintain and sustain competence in educating clinical and ancillary staff members.

Introduction:

As part of ongoing competence of staff development nurses, *individual ongoing self assessments* must be completed to assist in professional and personal development as an educator.

Key Action Tips:

- Self-assessment tools for the educator can reflect on the needs assessments of the learners.
- Review goals and objectives for educational programming to meet organizational objectives.

Example:

The staff development nurse educator can review the needs assessment of the learners that they are teaching to determine and prioritize needs as well as working to increase understanding of needs and modalities and techniques to encompass those needs. For example, when education of a new procedure or technique is required, the staff development nurse must connect with individuals and resources with which to increase skills and familiarity with the procedure, as well as the ability to troubleshoot issues that may arise.

Maintains Membership in Professional Organization

Definition:

The professional nursing staff educator holds memberships and actively participates in local and national organizations.

Introduction:

To maintain a high level of professional competence in clinical practice and to serve the role of staff educator, membership in local, state, and national organizations which support professional growth and development is encouraged.

Key Action Tips:

- Membership and active participation in the goals and objectives of professional organizations is recommended.
- Sharing of professional expertise and networking to find opportunities for shared experiences, goal-setting, and skill-building is mutually beneficial.
- Participation at the grassroots level is vital to finding solutions to educational issues.

Example:

Any of the following groups offer opportunities for networking with other staff educators in health care:

American Academy of Ambulatory Care Nursing – www.aaacn.org
- Offers monthly audio seminars (live or on CD-ROM) on a variety of topics related to ambulatory care nursing as well as a yearly conference with continuing education credits

American Nurses Association – www.nursingworld.org
- National nursing organization which certifies organizations that can provide continuing nursing education credits, and also contains the credentialing center for certification in nursing specialty areas

National Nurse Staff Development Organization – www.nnsdo.org
- Organization that promotes the professional nursing staff development nurse through encouragement of nursing research and continuing education programming; information on the nursing staff development certification is available on this site

Health Care Education Association – www.hcea-info.org
- Multidisciplinary professional organization of health educators that create instructional tools and resources for staff and patients from all venues, rural, urban, education, practice, and regulation; this organization offers a yearly continuing education conference on topics specific to staff and patient educators for continuing education units

National Health Education Group Web site of the United Kingdom –
http://www.nheg.org.uk/
- Annual conference each year for members
- Downloadable files on a variety of topics of interest to health educators

Serves as a Mentor

Definition:

The professional nursing staff educator serves as a mentor.

Introduction:

The role of the professional nursing staff educator is enhanced by the ability not only to teach specific skill sets to staff members, but also the ability to mentor and guide employees to meet their full potential, both personally and professionally. A mentor is a guide, leader, counselor, and trusted advisor.

Key Action Tips:

- Mentoring can impact the effectiveness of any educational endeavor as the teacher is equally as important to the learning process as is the learner.
- A mentor can build relationships with staff that will foster cooperation and collaborative relationships.

Example:

The nurse as mentor can develop and hone essential skills by reviewing the evidence on mentoring relationships and programs, and by integrating best practice into the mentoring opportunities within the organization. For example, a nurse educator can mentor staff to complete one-on-one "just in time" teaching of new policies, procedures, and processes.

Building a strong mentor presence can also encourage staff to mentor others within their work unit.

Conducts, Promotes, and Integrates Research into Practice

Definition:

The nurse as staff educator conducts, promotes, and integrates research into practice.

Introduction:

Evidence-based practice is crucial to maintaining a safe patient environment and to optimize positive health-sustaining outcomes. The staff educator can take a leadership role in training staff on the process of researching medical literature for best practice, and to individualize research within the practice that focuses on quality improvement efforts.

Key Action Tips:

- Evidence-based practice principles must be shared with staff at all levels in order to increase understanding of the process as well as to encourage cooperation and collaboration along all levels of staff members that are involved in the process.
- Review evidence-based practice books and journal articles.
- Work with local resources (e.g., medical librarians) to assist staff with reviewing the evidence and formulating study questions.

Example:

The staff educator can conduct mini-sessions on the key concepts of evidence-based practice and co-teach concepts with medical librarians and nurse researchers that are available at academic nursing programs. The educator can facilitate staff discussions of processes that need improvement, can assist with the literature search to see what the "evidence" is, and then to formulate a question that needs to be addressed and studied within the practice. This allows the nurse educator to cultivate evidence-based champions within the work unit that can then assist others.

Subscribes to Professional Journals

Definition:

The nurse as staff educator subscribes to professional journals and may lead a journal club.

Introduction:

With the exponential changes in health care delivery across all health care practices, the staff educator can take the lead in reviewing the medical literature for articles and then be a leader in sharing this information with staff for discussion.

Key Action Tips:

- The nurse educator must maintain professional memberships in health care organizations that will assist in maintaining professional standards of excellence and access to current best practices that are published in the medical literature.
- Collaborating with local health care medical libraries and building collaborative relationships with information sharing can be vital to this role.

Example:

The staff educator should be a leader within the organization to encourage administrative support for subscriptions to nursing/medical journals that can enhance practice. In addition, collaborations with local universities and medical libraries can assist staff to have the appropriate evidence available as needed for clinical practice applications.

Publishes in Professional Journals

Definition:

The nurse as staff educator publishes in professional journals.

Introduction:

The staff educator will be a leader within the health care practice in providing outcomes and publication of best practices, evidence-based endeavors, and educational principles, methods, and outcomes.

Key Action Tips:

- Writing for publication involves collaboration with editorial staff to determine type of articles within the publication.
- Find a mentor to assist with identification of issues and to edit manuscripts.
- Experience in writing can be obtained through writing workshops, working with published nursing authors, or collaborating with other members of the health care team.
- Review of manuscript writing guidelines for publication can assist the staff educator to focus the article to the readership of the journal.

Example:

- American Academy of Ambulatory Care Nursing (www.aaacn.org)
- *ViewPoint* newsletter, published bi-monthly
- Nursing journals (this is not an exhaustive list, but rather a point of reference):
  - *Advances in Nursing Science*
  - *AJN – American Journal of Nursing*
  - *Family and Community Health*
  - *The Health Care Manager*
  - *Journal for Nurses in Staff Development*
  - *Journal of Ambulatory Care Management*
  - *Holistic Nursing Practice*
  - *Journal of Nursing Care Quality*
  - *Nursing Educator*
  - *Nursing*

Develops Web-Based Instructional Tools

Definition:

The nurse as staff educator is an integral key to the development of not only classes, but also Web-based instructional modalities to fit the diverse learning needs of the health care practice.

Introduction:

With the advent of new Web 2.0 technologies and the diverse learning needs of staff members, the staff educator must embrace new and evolving interactive options for staff to impart vital information to staff members which can be accessed electronically and used in an interactive network.

Key Action Tips:

- Learn and practice with new delivery methods for imparting information, including, but not limited to, online interactive learning, RSS feeds, blogs, wikis, mash-ups, and the like.

Example:

Utilizing innovative technologies to enhance learning outside of the classroom setting, nurses can avail themselves of available classes and resources through continuing education courses, books, articles, and hands-on training with IT professionals. Use of Web 2.0 technologies and offering a class on their use could be a helpful way to mesh new advances into effective time-focused educational offerings for staff members.

Maintains Clinical Competency

Definition:

The nursing staff educator will maintain competence in clinical practice.

Introduction:

In order to be a confident, informed educator, the nursing staff educator will need to search out opportunities to continue to exhibit exemplary clinical practice within the practice setting.

Key Action Tips:

Work collegially with staff members to ensure clinical competence in procedures and processes of the practice while using nursing assessment skills to enhance patient care and positive patient outcomes. Attend appropriate educational offerings that focus on skill-building in clinical practice.

Example:

The nursing staff educator can retain, maintain, and grow clinical skills by working per diem shifts as appropriate. The nurse educator can also serve on the institutional Nursing Policy and Procedure Committee.

Pursues Continuing Education

Definition:

The nursing staff educator will continue to pursue continuing education opportunities through state/national nursing and/or management certifications and pursue additional academic preparation through undergraduate, graduate, post-graduate, and/or doctoral level studies.

Introduction:

Keeping abreast in a health care environment that changes and grows increasingly more complex is a primary challenge as well as an opportunity for the nurse educator. By working to be a role model and mentor for continued professional growth and development, the practice and its staff members will be able to provide ever more sophisticated, competent, and care-centered clinical practice to improve patient outcomes.

Key Action Tips:

- Serve on boards of schools of medical assistants, licensed practical/vocational, and registered nurses in a consultative role.
- Pursue continuing education from a variety of resources, such as online continuing education and conference attendance.
- Continue to build competencies in practice and education by pursuing post-graduate education in nursing or health-related fields.

Example:

The nurse staff educator could partner with local schools or universities to offer the practice site as an off campus location for degree seeking employees. In addition, the nurse staff educator could coordinate study groups that meet within the practice over lunch periods or before or after work to assist employees to find resources to assist them in their educational endeavors.

Reference

Wright, D. (2005). *The ultimate guide to competency assessment in health care* (3rd ed.). Minneapolis, MN: Creative Healthcare Management, Inc.

RESOURCES FOR THE NURSE TRANSITIONING TO AMBULATORY CARE

Catherine Liebau, MSN, RN

This guide is written for those nurses who are presently transitioning to an ambulatory care setting. There are 3 main objectives this guide will cover assisting with getting grounded in your ambulatory care role:

#1 — Identify clinical and administrative resources needed for successful ambulatory care nursing practice.

#2 — Describe the core knowledge needed for successful transition and practice of ambulatory care nursing.

#3 — Identify the competencies for an ambulatory care nurse.

What is Ambulatory Care Nursing?

It is a specialty practice setting that is fast-paced and unpredictable involving high volumes within a very short period of time. Ambulatory care nursing involves all age groups from many different cultures seeking assistance with their health maintenance and disease management. This type of specialty requires fast and focused assessments of patients/families to determine plan of care along with effective teaching skills supporting a reasonable translation to the patient/families.

What is Unique About Ambulatory Care?

Practice settings — Hospital-based or stand alone Emergency Departments, outpatient areas, and ambulatory surgery settings, urgent care, walk-in clinics, private practice provider clinics and offices.

Episodic — In that the care is given at the point of request or presentation and is only for that moment in time or of limited duration.

In person or via telephone — Telehealth, that is, supplying health care (health maintenance and disease management) using electronic technology such as the telephone and computer to assist with the management of care.

Workloads — Room assignments, physician practice assignments, staff assignments, call center or telephone assignments, or, finally, specific health maintenance or disease management assignments.

Appointment schedules — Patients seen on an appointment basis along with "walk-in" status.

Assessments — Can be done solely by the nurse seeing the patient as well as working through a family member to determine present health status/issue.

Independent — Use of the nursing process to determine patient need is done very independently. Nurses in this venue need to be confident in their knowledge and skills in order to be effective.

Team/Team Member — While needing to be able to function independently, the ambulatory care nurse needs to be aware of working within and feel part of a collaborative team.

Getting Started

Standards of Care

Ambulatory standards of care can be found in the following:

- AAACN *Telehealth Nursing Practice Administration and Practice Standards,* 4th Edition
- AAACN *Core Curriculum for Ambulatory Care Nursing,* 2nd Edition
- AAACN *Ambulatory Care Nursing Orientation and Competency Assessment Guide,* 2nd Edition
- AAACN *Scope and Standards of Practice for Professional Ambulatory Care Nursing,* 8th Edition

Core Clinical Knowledge

Core nursing knowledge needed to be effective in an ambulatory care venue is:

- Primary care — The knowledge of various health promotion, health maintenance, and disease management plans of care.
- Acute illness/injury — Plans of care regarding management of acute illnesses and injury. What can be managed and by whom.
- Chronic diseases — Plans of care for those patients with chronic illnesses and the awareness of integrating the plan within the patients' needs and abilities.
- Public health — Knowledge of management of communicable diseases along with patient, family, clinic impact. Ability to integrate public health initiatives with patient's plan of care.

Available Guidelines

General guidelines for illness/disease management and for health promotion and disease prevention are available on the Internet to assist with core clinical knowledge utilization and patient management in ambulatory care.

Illness and Disease Management:
- National Guideline Clearing House

Health Promotion/Disease Prevention:
- Guide to Community Prevention Services
- American Committee on Immunization Practices
- Immunization Action Coalition
- Partnership for Prevention
- Guide to Clinical Preventive Services – U.S. Preventive Services Task Force
  - Screening
  - Immunizations
  - Counseling
  - Preventive Medications

Telehealth

Ambulatory care nursing, compared to acute and long-term care, relies heavily on technology in their use of the nursing process. *Telehealth* is the term used to describe nursing use of technology and telecommunications in the coordination of and deliver of patient care. Some examples of the common technology used are:
- Telephone (headsets, Bluetooth® devices)
- Computers
  - EMR/MyChart
  - ePrescribe
  - Email
  - Fax
  - Internet (patient teaching/resources/staff education)

There are reference materials available to build telephone management skills appropriate for the ambulatory care setting:

American Academy of Ambulatory Care Nursing (AAACN). (2008). *ViewPoint, 30*(1-3). "Telehealth Trials and Triumphs" series by Kathy Koehne.
American Academy of Ambulatory Care Nursing (AAACN). (2009). *ViewPoint, 31*(5). Special issue on Telehealth Nursing.
American Telemedicine Association (ATA). (2008). *Telehealth nursing: A white paper developed and accepted by the Telehealth Nursing Special Interest Group.*
Espensen, M. (Ed.) (2009). *Telehealth nursing practice essentials.* Pitman, NJ: American Academy of Ambulatory Care Nursing.

Scope of Practice

Collaboration, in the ambulatory care setting, involves the employment of various levels of staff available to develop and execute a patient's plan of care. These various levels have their own "Scope of Practice" which needs to be acknowledged. In some cases, licensure is needed to provide certain patient care interventions. This becomes important when delegation of duties is necessary. It is important to check your local (State) Regulation and Licensing requirements to know what can be delegated, what is needed to delegate, and finally to whom to delegate.

Examples of different levels include, but are not limited to:
- Physician
- Nurse Practitioner
- Physician Assistant
- Registered Nurse
- Licensed Practical or Vocational Nurse
- Medical Assistant
- Medical Technician
- Administrative Assistant
- Schedulers
- Call Center staff

Competency Needs

In an effort to provide patients with an optimal plan of care, it is important for ambulatory care nurses to be competent in their skills. Some areas of skills are:

- Clinical knowledge and skill specific to the area of practice and population served
- Telephone triage/assessment
- Care/case management
- Collaboration in management and delivery of care
- Relationships with patients and families
- Health education
- Leadership
- Process/quality improvement

How Does Ambulatory Care Monitor or Measure Performance?

Similar to other nursing venues (i.e., acute care LTC), ambulatory care has performance measures for disease management and patient satisfaction. Here are common items being measured and trended in most ambulatory care venues.

Ambulatory Care Quality Measures

There are 2 domains that are measured in ambulatory care: clinical and non-clinical domain.

Clinical domains are:
- Immunization rates
- Health maintenance screening rates
- Disease-specific management
  - Cardiovascular
  - COPD
  - Diabetes
  - Hypertension
  - Mental health
  - Musculoskeletal

Non-clinical domains include:
- Access to care
  - Appointment availability
  - Telephone access
- Productivity indices
- Financial indices
- Satisfaction

Know what resources are available to provide the best patient interventions.

Here are some of the various patient intervention guidelines that are available:

Federal Resources (not an exhaustive list)
- U.S. Department of Health and Human Services
  - Administration on Aging (AoA)
  - Agency for Healthcare Research and Quality (AHRQ)
  - Centers for Disease Control and Prevention (CDC)
  - Centers for Medicare & Medicaid Services (CMS)
  - Food and Drug Administration (FDA)
  - Health Resources and Services Administration (HRSA)
  - Indian Health Services (IHS)
  - National Institutes of Health (NIH)
  - The National Women's Health Information Center (OWH)
  - Substance Abuse and Mental Health Services Administration (SAMHSA)
- National Institutes of Health
  - National Cancer Institute
  - National Center for Complementary and Alternative Medicine
  - National Heart, Lung, and Blood Institute
  - National Institute of Diabetes and Digestive and Kidney Disease
  - National Institutes of Health – Senior Health
  - National Institute on Aging
  - National Institute for Allergies and Infectious Diseases
  - National Library of Medicine
- U.S. Army Center for Health Promotion and Preventive Medicine
- U.S. Department of Veterans Affairs
  - National Center for Health Promotion and Disease Prevention
  - Office of Public Health and Environmental Hazards
  - Infection: Don't Pass It On

Non-Federal Resources (not an exhaustive list)

- Alcoholics Anonymous
- American Cancer Society
- American Dental Association
- American Diabetes Association
- American Heart Association
- American Lung Association
- American Red Cross
- American Social Health Association
- Cleveland Clinic
- Fifty-Plus Fitness Association
- Health Touch®
- Immunization Action Coalition
- Johns Hopkins
- Lupus Foundation
- Mayo Clinic
- National Center on Elder Abuse
- National Comprehensive Cancer Network
- National Sexual Violence Resource Center
- National Women's Resource Center
- Shape Up America
- Susan G. Komen for the Cure
- U.S. Army Hooah 4 Health
- Vanderbilt University
- Your Disease Risk

AAACN Resources

- *Ambulatory Care Nurse Staffing: An Annotated Bibliography*
- *Ambulatory Care Nursing Certification Review Course Syllabus*
- *Ambulatory Care Nursing Orientation and Competency Assessment Guide*, 2nd Edition
- *Ambulatory Care Nursing Review Questions*
- *Core Curriculum for Ambulatory Care Nursing*, 2nd Edition
- *Scope and Standards of Practice for Professional Ambulatory Care Nursing*, 8th Edition
- *Telehealth Nursing Practice Administration and Practice Standards*, 4th Edition
- *Telehealth Nursing Practice Essentials*
- *Telehealth Nursing Practice Resource Directory*

Bibliography

Del Monte, P. (n.d.). *New to ambulatory care nursing? What you need in your ambulatory care nursing toolkit*. PowerPoint presentation.

Appendices

Appendix A

Organizational Competency Assessment Tools

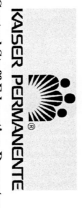

Tri Central Staff Education Department
Tri Central Service Area

Competency: Delegation of Tasks and Procedures

Scenario: You are the RN team leader for the "holding room" where ambulatory patients receive interventions and are monitored for up to 4 hours. Please exam the list below and check the task and procedures which you can legally delegate to an RN, LVN and medical assistant (MA) per the RN and LVN scope of practice regulations, the medical assistant laws and regulations, facility job descriptions and policies and procedures. All staff has had their competencies verified.

Task/Procedure	RN	LVN	MA
Insert an indwelling catheter			
Administer intravenous medication			
Use independent clinical judgment			
Perform patient assessment			
Perform and EKG			
Collect specimens, for e.g., urine, stool, sputum			
Take vital signs			
Accept verbal orders			
Administer an enema			
Obtain a throat culture			
Start an IV			
Use the title "Nurse"			
Conduct a neurological assessment			
Provide patient/family education			
Conduct a hearing screening test			
Use a urine specimen to perform a urine pregnancy test			
Perform a fingerstick and conduct blood sugar testing			
Discharge planning			
Assist with ambulation and transfer			
Count narcotics with a licensed person			
Perform venipuncture/Withdraw blood			
Interpret and document Tuberculin test results			

Name: _____

Department: _____   Date: _____

Reprinted with permission from Kaiser Permanente, Tricentral Staff Education Department

FN: Delegation of Task/Procedures
LJFlint, RN
1/05

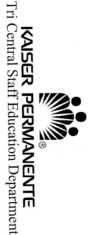

KAISER PERMANENTE®
Tri Central Staff Education Department

Tri Central Service Area

Competency: Environmental Management

Environmental Management Tasks: Utilize the attached diagram of the T. Ward Family Medicine Facility in which you work, to complete the following:

1. Using an asterisk symbol (*), mark the location of all the fire extinguishers directly on the diagram.

2. Using a happy face symbol (☺), mark the location of all the fire "pull" alarms directly on the diagram.

3. Using a heart symbol (♥), mark the location of all the automatic external defibrillators (AEDs) directly on the diagram.

4. Using the symbol (W/C), mark the location of the wheelchair accessible scale directly on the diagram.

5. Using the symbol (EP), mark the location of the emergency preparedness equipment and supplies, directly on the diagram.

6. Code orange identifies what type of emergent issue?

    a. _____

7. Specify the circumstances which would lead you to have a Code yellow paged.

    b. _____

8. What number do you dial to initiate a:

    a. Code Orange _____
    b. Code Red _____
    c. Code Blue _____
    d. Code Yellow _____

9. You are the only nurse assigned to the holding room today, but fortunately the workload has been manageable and pleasant. As you walk toward Raphael to assess his vital signs you are thrown to the floor by a large and forceful explosion. You have no idea where the explosion initiated but heavy caustic smoke has begun to rapidly enter the holding area from the south side of the room. You are bleeding heavily from a deep scalp laceration probably caused by flying glass. You have the following three patients in the holding room on gurneys:

a. Raphael, a 6 month old infant with a fever of 104°F for whom you were providing cooling measures. He is there with his 26 year old mother, Jane.

b. Mr. William Caldwell, 44 year old wheelchair active, paraplegic is in for stool impaction removal and cleansing enemas.

c. Mrs. Bessie Martin a 76 year Alzheimer patient who was dropped off by her daughter because Bessie's blood sugar was 50 this morning. Mrs. Martin is receiving intravenous therapy intervention and blood sugar monitoring. She has received medication to sedate her during therapy.

The code for an internal disaster with subsequent evacuation has been paged. **Use the facility diagram as a point of reference.** What is your course of action? Please be specific.

FN: Environmental Management
LJFlint

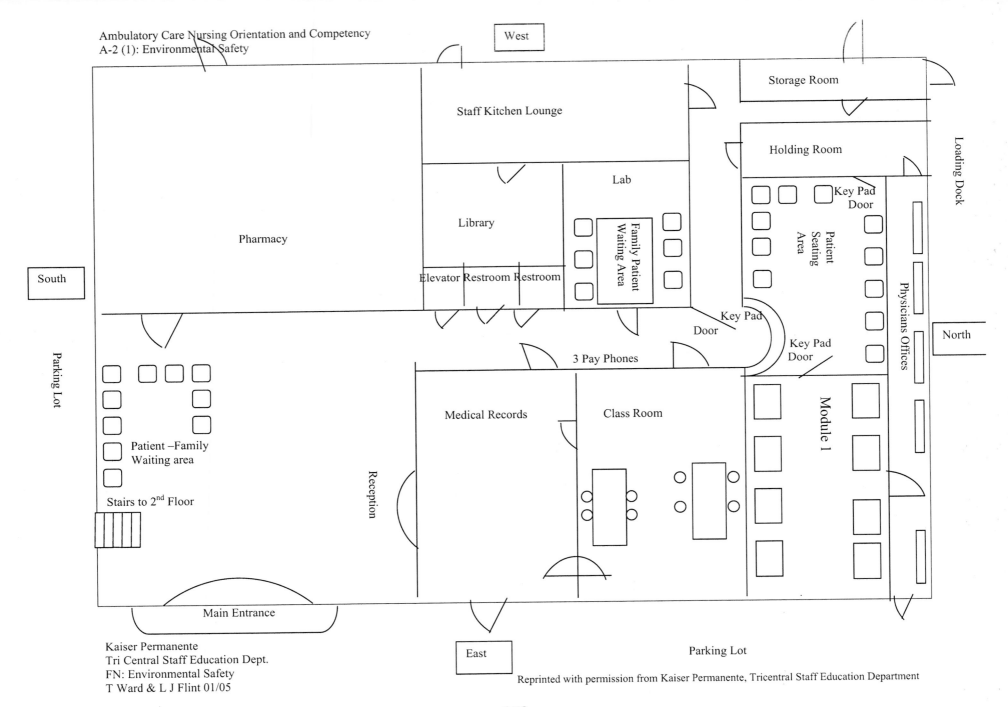

West

Storage Room

Staff Kitchen Lounge

Loading Dock

Holding Room

Lab

Key Pad Door

Library

Patient Seating Area

Pharmacy

Family Patient Waiting Area

South

Elevator Restroom Restroom

Physicians Offices

Key Pad Door

North

Door

Key Pad Door

3 Pay Phones

Parking Lot

Patient –Family Waiting area

Reception

Medical Records

Class Room

Module 1

Stairs to 2nd Floor

Main Entrance

East

Parking Lot

Kaiser Permanente
Tri Central Staff Education Dept.
FN: Environmental Safety
T Ward & L J Flint 01/05

Reprinted with permission from Kaiser Permanente, Tricentral Staff Education Department

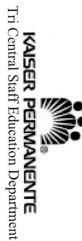

KAISER PERMANENTE

Tri Central Staff Education Department

Tri Central Service Area

Competency: Ethics

Scenario: You and Mae are bosom buddies who have shared an apartment for the past 5 years. The two of you met while attending nursing school and now work for the same employer; a very large and busy family practice facility. You are the newly appointed facility nursing supervisor for the evening shift. Mae works the day shift as a staff RN in the "holding room" where patients receive intervention and are monitored up to 4 hours. You are glad to be on the evening shift so your new role does not place you in the direct position of supervising your best friend.

Over the weekend while preparing a barbecue to celebrate your promotion with friends, Mae blurts out that she is so relieved that the work week is over. "I nearly killed a patient". Taken back by her statement and upon inquiring further about Mae's remarks she states, "I have never been so scared in my life. I gave a patient twice the amount of narcotic ordered by mistake, but I signed for the ordered amount on the chart and narcotic record. I was so nervous I didn't take a break or have lunch so I could constantly monitor him. Thank goodness he was a very large man as I believe his size helped to keep his vital signs stable. I was so relieved when the physician examined him and discharged him home I almost wet my pants. What a relief to get this off of my chest. Now I can really enjoy the party for your promotion".

1. Define "ethical dilemma".

2. According to your definition does this scenario present as an ethical dilemma?

3. What ethical principles, if any are implicated in this scenario?

4. What, if any legal issues are presented in the scenario?

5. What are your options?

6. Which option would you choose if you found yourself in this situation and why? Please be specific.

FN: Ethical Dilemma
LJFlint, RN
1/05

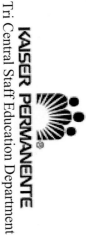

KAISER PERMANENTE

Tri Central Staff Education Department

Tri Central Service Area

Competency: Informatics and HIPAA

Background: Health Insurance Portability and Accountability Act (HIPAA), a commitment to patient information security is also a requirement of federal law. Everyone in your family medicine facility has completed HIPAA training as well as 12 hours of computer fundamentals for the organization's new automated medical record system which has gone "live". As an RN you have completed an additional 4 hours of HIPAA and informatics training with emphasis on serving as an expert resource for staff.

Scenario: Your assignment as a supervising RN requires facility roaming (receptionist station, nurse visit, call center, exam rooms, triage, medical records, etc.), necessitating frequent computer access to patient data and opportunities to evaluate staffs' computer proficiency and adherence of HIPAA mandates for informatics. Identify the 4 critical intercessions you and your staff must consistently employ to prevent inappropriate access to patients' automated medical records. <u>Please be specific.</u>

1.

2.

3.

4.

FN: HIPAA Informatics
LJFlint/DHughes
1/05

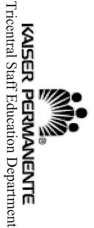

KAISER PERMANENTE
Tricentral Staff Education Department

Tri-Central Service Area

Competency: Informatics Application

Assignment: You have 45 minutes to complete this assignment. At the "dummy" computer workstation, demonstrate your informatics acumen by completing the clinical task listed below.

Print out and submit the completed assignments to the informatics application instructor for analysis and competency verification

Completed task are equally assessed for the quality of your documentation entry.

Clinical Informatics Task:

1. Print out the patient instruction form for Maggie Apple on preventing urinary tract infections

2. Open and print out an encounter and use a "SmartText" to document the ear wash procedure you completed on Mary Smith.

3. Initiate and print out laboratory orders for a throat culture, CBC, urinalysis and chest x-ray for Peter Paul.

4. Jan Johnson is a new patient to Kaiser Permanente. Open a new encounter, document and print out the following data for Jan: temperature, 98.6° F, pulse 64, respirations 16, blood pressure 165/90, weight 240 lbs., height 6'0, and fingerstick blood sugar 180. Allergic to Aspirin, dogs, and chamomile.

5. Dr. Adon has ordered an influenza vaccine for Jan Johnson. Print out his order, a listing of Jan's allergies and your documentation of the administered medication.

6. The nurse practitioner closed the encounter for Kenya Amari before you had a chance to finish documenting. Create and print out an addendum stating Ms. Amari states "I will attend the Diabetic management class on August 4, 2005".

7. You are on the telephone with Jan Johnson. She can't remember what her laboratory blood glucose result was and ask that you check for her as she keeps a record of all her results. Print the laboratory result and document on and print the telephone encounter.

8. Create a message indicating the department staff meeting for 1200 tomorrow has been cancelled. It will be rescheduled, date to be announced. Send and print out a copy of the message you send to, Barbara Jones, Juan Garcia, Maxine Chusak, and Florence Nightingale.

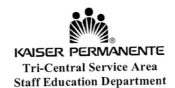

KAISER PERMANENTE

Tri-Central Service Area

Staff Education Department

Accurate Blood Pressure Measurement Competency Audit ©

Audit event #	1	2	3	4	5	6	7	8	9	10	TOTAL # of +'s	Compliance %
Date:												
1. Member Position												
☐ Erect, back supported												
☐ Both feet on floor												
☐ Quiet												
2. Cuff												
☐ Bare arm												
☐ 80/40 rule												
☐ 1 ½ inches above elbow												
☐ Snug, allowing one finger insertion												
☐ Arm extended at heart level and supported												
3. Blood Pressure												
☐ Ask member about their "usual" BP reading												
☐ Inflates manual cuff 30mm above member's "usual BP reading"												
☐ Repeats BP reading in same arm, following a 1-2 minute rest period, if initial reading is 140/90 or higher												
☐ Documentation reflects initial and repeat reading including time of each.												
Total # of +'s per event												

Legend: + = Yes   Ø = No

Baldwin Park HTN Committee

FN: Audit BP Measurement

LJFlint

2/12/04

Revised 12/04

162

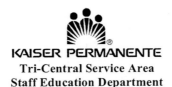

KAISER PERMANENTE®
Tri-Central Service Area
Staff Education Department

Accurate Blood Pressure Measurement Competency Audit ©

Individual Audit Event Comments:

1.	
2.	
3.	
4.	
5.	
6.	
7.	
8.	
9.	
10.	

Employee Name and Title: _____ Department: _____

Auditor Name and Title: _____ Date completed tool submitted to Department Administrator: _____

Dept. Administrator Name and Title: _____

Plan of Action including target dates and re-evaluation:

_____

_____

_____

_____

Baldwin Park HTN Committee
FN: Audit BP Measurement
LJFlint
2/12/04
Revised 12/04

Reprinted with permission from Kaiser Permanente, Tricentral Staff Education

163

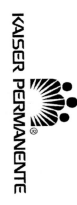

Tri-Central Service Area
Staff Education Department

DOCUMENTATION COMPETENCY CHART AUDIT TOOL
FOR MEDICAL OFFICE VISITS©

Medical Center: ___ Baldwin Park ___ Bellflower ___ South Bay

Medical Office: _____ Module: _____

Patient's Medical Record Number: _____ Date: _____

Auditor's Name/Title: _____

Documentation Audit Criteria for Medical Office Visit	Yes	No	N/A	Comments
1. Document/page/form audited contains patient's name, medical record #, DOB.				
2. Documentation written in black ink.				
3. Form dated with month, day and year				
4. Legible documentation. (Trouble reading the entry, then mark 'No).				
5. Entries spelled correctly.				
6. Approved abbreviations used. (Refer to MCW approved abbreviation list).				
7. Data requested complete- No blank lines.				
8. Abnormal data circled.				
9. Entry signed with author's first initial, full last name and job title. Full first and last name along + job title acceptable.				
10. Documentation errors legally corrected: ◆ Single line drawn through mistake. ◆ "Error" written above mistake. ◆ Author's initials located next to the word "error." (Date and time next to author's initials is recommended but optional).				
11. Chart contains face sheet, health maintenance record, diabetic flow sheet (if applicable)				
Total Number of "Yes", "No" and "N/A" Responses				

Reprinted with permission from Kaiser Permanente, Tricentral Staff Education Department

FN: SLM Documentation Audit Tool
R. Haynes and L.J.Flint
5/13/04

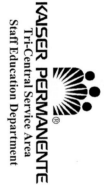

KAISER PERMANENTE®
Tri-Central Service Area
Staff Education Department

DOCUMENTATION COMPETENCY AUDIT TOOL FOR MEDICAL OFFICE VISITS: Tabulation Summary Report ©

Audit Criteria	Tally # of "No" Responses for each chart audited	Total # of "No's"	*Percentage
1. Document/page/form audited contains patient's name, medical record #, DOB.			
2. Documentation written in black ink.			
3. Form dated with month, day and year			
4. Legible documentation. (Trouble reading the entry, then mark "No).			
5. Entries spelled correctly.			
6. Approved abbreviations used. (Refer to MCW approved abbreviation list).			
7. Data requested complete- No blank lines.			
8. Abnormal data circled (Vital Signs).			
9. Entry signed with author's first initial, full last name and job title. Full first and last name along + job title acceptable.			
10. Documentation errors legally corrected: ◆ Single line drawn through mistake. ◆ "Error" written above mistake. ◆ Author's initials located next to the word "error." (Date and time next to author's initials is recommended but optional).			
11. Chart contains face sheet, health maintenance record, diabetic flow sheet (if applicable)		Grand Total of "No" Responses:	

*Percentage is obtained by dividing total # of "no" responses in column 3 by the total # of completed audit charts. For example 10 "no's" divided by a total of 75 charts audited…10/75 = 13%. Next subtract 13% from 100% = 87% compliance rate for the specified audit criteria.

Audit Criteria with Highest Number of "No" Responses (Top 3)

1. _____
2. _____
3. _____

Analysis/Findings:

_____

_____

_____

_____

_____

Plan of Action Including Target Dates: Focus on top 3 "No" responses above

_____

_____

_____

_____

_____

_____

_____

_____

Top Twenty Non - Approved Charting Abbreviations:

1. _____   11. _____
2. _____   12. _____
3. _____   13. _____
4. _____   14. _____
5. _____   15. _____
6. _____   16. _____
7. _____   17. _____
8. _____   18. _____
9. _____   19. _____
10. _____   20. _____

FN: Tabulation Summary Audit
LJFlint
10/27/04

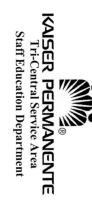

KAISER PERMANENTE®
Tri-Central Service Area
Staff Education Department

Medical Center: __ Baldwin Park __ Bellflower __ Harbor City

Medical Office: _____ Module(s): _____

Total Number of Documentation Audit Charts Completed: _____

Names/titles of staff participating in process:

_____

_____

_____

Report Submitted by: _____ **Date:** _____

Reprinted with permission from Kaiser Permanente, Tricentral Staff Education Department

FN: Tabulation Summary Audit

Appendix B

Nursing Practice Competencies

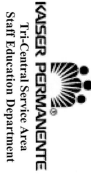

KAISER PERMANENTE
Tri-Central Service Area
Staff Education Department

URINE PREGNANCY TEST©

Name: _____ Unit: _____ Date: _____

This skill applies to	RCP	RN	LVN II	LVN	NA/CNA	MA/CA	Tech. Partner	MD, RNP, PA	Others (Specify)
	No	Yes	Yes	Yes	No	Yes	No		

COMPETENCY VALIDATION

	CRITICAL THINKING		PSYCHOMOTOR (SKILL)			INTERPERSONAL	
	Rating	MSE	Date	Rating	MSE	Date	Rating	MSE	Date

PSYCHOMOTOR (SKILL)

1. Collects and labels urine sample with patient's name and medical record number

2. Verifies prior to test:
   (a) Documented laboratory quality control
   (b) Proper storage and expiration date of test kit

3. Performs test:
   (a) Verbalizes and demonstrates appropriate sample volume and application
   (b) Accurately interprets test results within allotted timeframe
   (c) Documents results on the patient's record

4. States criteria for valid test results

5. Verbalizes limitations of procedure and demonstrates troubleshooting in the event of an error

CRITICAL THINKING

1. What actions do you initiate when a blue line appears in the control window?

2. Mrs. Crowder submits a non-refrigerated urine specimen she collected 5 hours ago. You have a physician order for pregnancy testing. Describe your actions and rationale.

INTERPERSONAL (Diversity, Age Specific, Customer Service)

1. Describe 5 considerations you will apply when approaching and preparing 52 year old, Suen Chang for a urine pregnancy test?

- Procedure integrates and adheres to standard precautions, and patient safety and education standards.

- **References:**
  a.) Pacific Biotech, Inc., 08/00. Subsidiary of QUIDEL Corporation, San Diego, CA 92121.
  b.) Baldwin Park policy and procedures # 2650 and 2650.50

LJ Flint 1/05

Validated By: _____ **Title** _____ **Date:** _____

Skill Rating:

☐ *Novice*   ☐ Independent   ☐ Expert   ☐ *Not Met*

Special Note:

1. **Documentation is required for Novice or Not Met skill rating.**
2. **Specify measurable action(s) to guide the employee at minimum, to an independent rating.**
2. **Include target for completion of action plan including date and time to re-validate staff.**

Comments:

Action Plan:

Skill Rating Guidelines/Definitions - Baldwin Park P/P #4028.00:

Novice............ Can undertake skill but must be supervised/checked by a validator. Completes skill elements but beyond time frames. Requires assistance from the appropriate persons. May need to review the P/P but needs minimal prompting

Independent........ Undertakes the skill easily, readily, with time frames, without any assistance or prompting

Expert............ Can teach the skill and is a resource to others. Has in-depth understanding of the skill and problems solving. Works at maximum level of efficiency and confidence. Is a trainer or validator in the department for the skill.

Not Met........... Cannot undertake the skill. Does not or is unable to perform the skill despite following P/P or given assistance/prompting. Continues to make the same mistakes.

Method of Skill Evaluation (MSE) - Baldwin Park P/P #4028.00:

RS-Routine Supervision (preferred method of choice in direct patient care setting)
RD - Return Demonstration
VO - Validator Observation
WA - Written Assessment
CA - Chart Audit
PFB - Patient Feedback
V - Verbalize Response/Understanding
PCS - Patient Care Scenarios
NO - Not Observed (only if not a critical element of the job)

Kelsey-Seybold Clinic
Patient Care Competency Review for LVN /RN

Name:_____ SS #_____   **Chart Audit Score** _____

Site:_____   **Medication Test Score**_____

Dept:_____   **Telephone Audit Score**_____

<u>Score</u> each area * **1 needs additional learning**   ***Performance Improvement Plan required for a Score of less**

                     2 meets standard of skill   **than 90% (on med test or phone audit) 80% (on chart audit)**

                     3 exceeds proficiency

                     NA skill is never performed in this position   **(Refer to instructors guide sheet for skills standard)**

Score	Patient Care Skills Check list	Date and Signature
	Vital Signs B/P, pulse, respiration, temperature, height, weight .Performs accurately and documents correctly	
	Respiratory Care Can perform peak flow test. Can apply pulse oximeter correctly Can apply O2 via mask or cannula.	
	Cath and /or Sterile fields Can set up and maintain sterile field. Or may demonstrate proper sterile technique for male and female catheterization.Appropiately cares for instruments. Actively uses universal precautions.Gloving,handwashing demonstrated between patients and before assisting with sterile procedures.	
	Pedi measurements : (temp, FOC, length, weight, graphing on growth chart	
	Lab handling cultures, pathology, PAP, urine, Hemocult, body fluid cytology, spinal fluid. Demonstrates or verbalizes proper handling	
	Code Blue Use of cart equipment, knows who and how to call for code team. Current CPR ,attends mock code and inservice.	
	Infection Control Station cleaning, biohazard clean up products, PPE, biohazard waste disposal.	
	Waive Testing Urine Dip, Pregnancy test, Blood Glucose, and Hemocult, accurately performs waive testing using appropriate Quality Controls. Documents results. Uses proper protective equipment (**circle ones that apply to this position**)	
	Medication Administration Uses 5 rights to accurately administer and monitor response to medication. Demonstrates proper technique for IM, SQ, ID, Rectal, oral ,and inhalant administration..	
	IV insertion and maintenance Demonstrates insertion on peripheal IV, set up , calculate drip rate, chart and discontinue	
	Comments	

Projects:AAACN:Books:Competencies:B-2 PT CARE SKILLS C#516AC.DOC

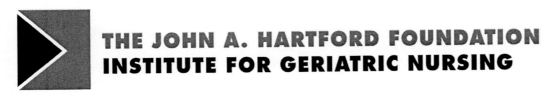

THE JOHN A. HARTFORD FOUNDATION
INSTITUTE FOR GERIATRIC NURSING

AMERICAN ACADEMY OF
AMBULATORY CARE NURSING
(AAACN)

Competency: Care of Adult 65 years +
AMBULATORY CARE

Method of Evaluation Key:

Knowledge: **T**-Test/Self Learning Module, **S**-Simulation/Scenario, **V**-Verbalizes Understanding

Skills and Behavior: **O**-Direct Observation, **MR**-Medical Record Audit, **RD**-Return Demonstration, **NA**=Not Applicable

COMPETENCIES	Self Evaluation By Employee			Validation of Competency	
	No Prior Experience	Needs to Review	Can Perform	Date Preceptor/Evaluator Signature Print Name	Evaluation Method (See Key Above)
1. **COMMUNICATION:** For older adults, demonstrate knowledge, skills and behavior of best practices in order to:					
Use communication strategies to meet patients' needs					
Assure participation in decision making: advance directives, health care proxy, DNR, informed consent, end-of-life care					
Assess barriers (drug interactions, dementia, delirium, disease states, depression) that impact patients' understanding of information, following directions and making needs known					
Assess impact of any decreased visual and/or auditory acuity.					
Educate patients and their families about the need to come prepared to ambulatory care visits. For example, bring all medications, write down questions prior to visits.					
Demonstrate familiarity w/adaptive devices (hearing aid, listenator)					

AAACN 03/23/04

Example: B3 Clinical nursing Competency

Competency: Care of Adult 65 years + *AMBULATORY CARE*

Method of Evaluation Key:

Knowledge: **T**-Test/Self Learning Module, **S**-Simulation/Scenario, **V**-Verbalizes Understanding

Skills and Behavior: O-Direct Observation, **MR**-Medical Record Audit, **RD**-Return Demonstration, **NA**=Not Applicable

COMPETENCIES	Self Evaluation By Employee			Validation of Competency	
	No Prior Experience	Needs to Review	Can Perform	Date Preceptor/Evaluator Signature Print Name	Evaluation Method (See Key Above)
Assess the relation of diversity to variations in the aging process (e.g. gender, race, culture, economic status, ethnicity, and sexual orientation).					
Ask permission for family or caregiver to attend appointment with patient; if no one is available ask, permission to telephone family member or caregiver.					
2. <u>PHYSIOLOGICAL AND PSYCHOLOGICAL AGE CHANGES</u>: For older adults, demonstrate knowledge, skills and behavior of best practices in order to:					
Intervene to address changes in temperature, BUN and creatinine					
Assess cognitive status for delirium, dementia and/or depression. Use standardized scale to assess:					
Establish baseline Mental Status (e.g., Mini Mental Status Examination - MMSE) to aid in diagnosis and changes from baseline.					
Depression (e.g., Geriatric Depression Scale - GDS *Short Form*)					
Use organization's established criteria for management of polypharmacy					
Intervene to eliminate or sharply curtail adverse events associated with medications, diagnostic or therapeutic procedures, nosocomial infections or environmental stressors					

Example: B3 Clinical nursing Competency

Competency: Care of Adult 65 years +
AMBULATORY CARE

COMPETENCIES	Self Evaluation By Employee			Validation of Competency	
	No Prior Experience	Needs to Review	Can Perform	Date Preceptor/Evaluator Signature Print Name	Evaluation Method (See Key Above)
3. **PAIN:** For older adults, demonstrate knowledge, skills and behavior of best practices in order to:					
Assess pain in cognitively impaired patients using valid and reliable self-report instruments and/or observations of patient behaviors (agitation, withdrawal, vocalizations, facial response/grimaces) *					
Intervene for the cognitively impaired when assessment is inconclusive and pain is to be expected					
* assessment & management of pain in cognitively intact older patients is no different than all patients					
4. **SKIN INTEGRITY:** For older adults, demonstrate knowledge, skills and behavior of best practices in order to:					
Assess the risk of skin breakdown using a standardized scale (e.g., Braden Scale)					
Educate about established criteria to implement appropriate bathing, choice of skin products, and positioning					
5. **FUNCTIONAL STATUS:** For older adults, demonstrate knowledge, skills and behavior of best practices in order to:					
Overall function:					
Demonstrates within care plan appropriate intervention to promote function in response to change in activities of daily living(ADL) and instrumental activities of daily living(IADL)					

176

Competency: Care of Adult 65 years +
AMBULATORY CARE

Method of Evaluation Key:
Knowledge: **T**-Test/Self Learning Module, **S**-Simulation/Scenario, **V**-Verbalizes Understanding
Skills and Behavior: **O**-Direct Observation, **MR**-Medical Record Audit, **RD**-Return Demonstration, **NA**=Not Applicable

COMPETENCIES	Self Evaluation By Employee			Validation of Competency	
	No Prior Experience	Needs to Review	Can Perform	Date Preceptor/Evaluator Signature Print Name	Evaluation Method (See Key Above)
Use assistive devices and suggest or initiate referral to appropriate therapies (OT, PT, ST) to promote and maintain optimal function					
Assess functional status using standardized scale (e.g. SF-36, SF-12) or based on regulatory requirements					
Administer "Get up and Go" (GUG) Test for ambulatory care (Mathias, S. et al. 1986)					
Urinary incontinence:					
Identify and refer to appropriate clinican recent onset of urinary incontinence (UI)					
Document rational for use of indwelling catheters other than in specified clinical situations(e.g., stage III/IV pressure ulcers, monitored acutely ill patients, urinary retention not manageable by other means)					
Assess urinary incontinence using current guideline					
Assess use of pads and/or depends					
Discuss cleaners and barriers, where to purchase these supplies, and cost of these supplies; if Medicaid, where to fax prescription					
Nutrition/Hydration:					
Use organization's established criteria to identify high risk patients for nutritional/fluid deficit					

Competency: Care of Adult 65 years +
AMBULATORY CARE

COMPETENCIES	Self Evaluation By Employee			Validation of Competency	
	No Prior Experience	Needs to Review	Can Perform	Date Preceptor/Evaluator Signature Print Name	Evaluation Method (See Key Above)
Intervene to address barriers to nutritional/fluid adequacy (e.g., difficulty with chewing & swallowing, alterations in hunger and thirst, inability to self feed & capacity of others to feed)					
Educate on nutritional supplements (Ensure, Boost, store brands, carnation instant breakfast) and how many to drink daily					
Educate the patient and/or family about the need to document weekly weight					
Falls, injuries, and safety precautions :					
Use a valid and reliable measure of fall risk assessment					
Use the organization's established falls prevention protocol					
Discuss home safety issues, such as burns, driving ability etc. and evaluation of home if applicable and available					
6. RESTRAINTS: For older adults, demonstrate knowledge, skills and behavior of best practices in order to:					
Document discussion of the use of a physical restraint(Posey, mitts, chairs with fixed trays, sheets, side rails)					
Document behavior of patient who is physically restrained					
Intervene to eliminate or sharply curtail the use of physical restraints (e.g. alternate strategies to prevent falls, to prevent treatment interference, and to manage agitated and/or combative behavior)					

AAACN 03/23/04

Competency: Care of Adult 65 years +
AMBULATORY CARE

Method of Evaluation Key:

Knowledge: **T**-Test/Self Learning Module, **S**-Simulation/Scenario, **V**-Verbalizes Understanding

Skills and Behavior: **O**-Direct Observation, **MR**-Medical Record Audit, **RD**-Return Demonstration, **NA**=Not Applicable

COMPETENCIES	Self Evaluation By Employee			Validation of Competency	
	No Prior Experience	Needs to Review	Can Perform	Date Preceptor/Evaluator Signature Print Name	Evaluation Method (See Key Above)
7. **ELDER ABUSE:** For older adults, demonstrate knowledge, skills and behavior of best practices in order to:					
Demonstrate knowledge applicable to mandated reporting for suspected abuse					
Demonstrate knowledge of risk factors and types of abuse/neglect					
Identify agencies that can assist with abuse and/or neglect					
Use organization's established criteria to identify elder abuse					
8. **DISCHARGE PLANNING:** For older adults, demonstrate knowledge, skills and behavior of best practices in order to:					
Educate the patient and/or family about the need to verify follow-up appointment with primary care provider (PCP) in 7 to 10 days after hospitalization or ER visit (if applicable).					
Educate patient/families to bring records from hospital/ER visits to PCP appointments.					
Assess role of caregiver and availability of resources and resource systems for caregiver support (if applicable).					

AAACN 03/23/04

Example: B3 Clinical nursing Competency

Competency: Care of Adult 65 years +
AMBULATORY CARE

Method of Evaluation Key:

Knowledge: **T**-Test/Self Learning Module, **S**-Simulation/Scenario, **V**-Verbalizes Understanding

Skills and Behavior: **O**-Direct Observation, **MR**-Medical Record Audit, **RD**-Return Demonstration, **NA**=Not Applicable

COMPETENCIES	Self Evaluation By Employee			Validation of Competency	
	No Prior Experience	Needs to Review	Can Perform	Date Preceptor/Evaluator Signature Print Name	Evaluation Method (See Key Above)
Transmit timely and complete information to patient/family, home care/ skilled nursing facility (e.g. minimal data elements include diagnoses and medications, including dose & last dose taken)					
Provide patient education materials that are legible, printed clearly and at appropriate level of medical literacy					
Refer for evaluation of the need for special resources for transition to home (e.g., Meals on Wheels, adaptive devices, etc.)					

Adapted with permission for Ambulatory Care by the American Academy of Ambulatory Care Nursing (AAACN) in collaboration with the John A. Hartford Foundation for Geriatric Nursing

23-Mar-04

The John A. Hartford Foundation For Geriatric Nursing
New York University, The Steinhardt School of Education, Division of Nursing
246 Greene Street, 6th floor, New York, NY 10003
tel:212-998-9018 fax:212-995-4770 email:hartford.ign@nyu.edu
web site:http://www.hartfordign.org

TELEHEALTH NURSING PRACTICE ORIENTATION COMPETENCIES

EMPLOYEE: _____ HIRE DATE: _____ PRECEPTOR: _____

Orientation Competencies	Novice/Expert Weight Factor		Tested	Observed		Exceeds Expectations	Meets Expectations	Does Not Meet Expectations
1. Demonstrates appropriate and efficient use of department specific equipment/ software necessary to perform role (multi-feature telephones, automatic call distribution (ACD), keyboard skills, Windows and call processing software, modem, fax, copier, etc.								
1.1. Demonstrate knowledge and skill to correctly log onto telephone system, initiate and complete transfers, paging, conference calls, call parking, call hold, log after call work in not ready made, long distance call, and log off ACD.								
1.2. Demonstrate knowledge and skill to navigate in Windows environment such as Microsoft Windows or other operating system								
1.3. Demonstrate data entry skill at a minimum of 30-35 wpm without typos.								
1.4. Using the call processing software, demonstrate knowledge and skill in: a) accessing functions b) entering and saving data c) moving efficiently between functions								
1.5 Using the call processing software, demonstrates: a) registration of the caller/patient b) physician referrals/appointment for caller c) physician-to-physician referrals								

TELEHEALTH NURSING PRACTICE ORIENTATION COMPETENCIES

EMPLOYEE: _____ **HIRE DATE:** _____ **PRECEPTOR:** _____

Orientation Competencies	Novice/Expert Weight Factor	Tested	Observed	Exceeds Expectations	Meets Expectations	Does Not Meet Expectations
2. Able to express clearly the nature and scope of services for the program, including but not limited to: 2.1. Define mission of service. 2.2. Describe client populations served by program. 2.3. Following process/call management guides specific to the client population. 2.4. Comply with nursing scope of practice for state where nurse resides/service originates. 3. Demonstrates positive telephone interaction skills as evidenced by: 3.1. Courteousness (identifies self, refers to caller by name, pleasant tone of voice, allow caller to express issue, etc.) 3.2. Speaks directly to individual with symptoms whenever possible. 3.3 Asks open-ended questions to identify actual or potential health problems. 3.4 Restates problem to verify congruency with caller's perception. 3.5 Uses lay terminology when providing explanations and instructions. 3.6. Focuses conversations for goal-directed, time-limited communication. 3.7. Offers caller opportunity to express any concerns/ problems before ending call.						

Proposed compJuly.com
Carole Becker, MS, RN
07/12/99

07/08/99

TELEHEALTH NURSING PRACTICE ORIENTATION COMPETENCIES

EMPLOYEE: _____ **HIRE DATE:** _____ **PRECEPTOR:** _____

Orientation Competencies	Novice/Expert Weight Factor	Tested	Observed	Exceeds Expectations	Meets Expectations	Does Not Meet Expectations

4. Complies with call management standards:
   4.1. Answers phone on or before 3 rings 85% of all calls handled.
   4.2. Responds to highest priority call in queue.
   4.3. Call back to caller leaving message within 30 minutes 85% of all calls handled.
   4.4. Maintains professional composure in high stress, emotional situations.
   4.5. Maintains confidentiality of all interactions.
   4.6. Manages 85% of population specific calls within the LOC benchmarks established by call center.
 	
5. Demonstrates thorough knowledge of the program's identified top 20 triage guidelines.
 	
6. Using nursing knowledge and skill, manages clinical calls using the nursing process:
   6.1. Assesses life-threatening or crisis situations at onset of a call and manages referral to EMS.
   6.2. Record the caller-presenting problem; include specific quote of caller perception of the problem, its onset, severity, duration and any other current symptoms.						

Proposed compJuly.com
Carole Becker, MS, RN
07/12/99

07/08/99

TELEHEALTH NURSING PRACTICE ORIENTATION COMPETENCIES

EMPLOYEE: _____ **HIRE DATE:** _____ **PRECEPTOR:** _____

Orientation Competencies	Novice/Expert Weight Factor		Tested	Observed		Exceeds Expectations	Meets Expectations	Does Not Meet Expectations
6.3. Assesses and documents relevant clinical profile of the caller for current situation, including diagnosed health problems, recent infections/exposure, recent procedures/surgeries, current prescribed/OTC medications, known allergies/reactions, health risks.								
6.4. Demonstrates critical thinking by assessing covert as well as overt parameters relevant to the needs of the caller.								
6.5. Establishes priorities. Able to reprioritize as situation requires.								
6.6. Based on assessed information, accurately determines the most appropriate triage guideline for the situation for 95% of all calls.								
6.7. Follows organization approved triage guidelines, with each call (if available) 100% of all calls.								
6.8. Follows organization defined procedure for managing a symptom-based call when no triage guideline is included in the clinical database.								
6.9. Uses additional references when needed to meet the needs of the caller.								
6.10. Demonstrates knowledge of organization and community resources available to meet caller needs.								
6.11. Utilizes clinical assessment of caller variables to maintain appropriateness of disposition (defined								

TELEHEALTH NURSING PRACTICE ORIENTATION COMPETENCIES

EMPLOYEE: _____ **HIRE DATE:** _____ **PRECEPTOR:** _____

Orientation Competencies	Novice/Expert Weight Factor	Tested	Observed	Exceeds Expectations	Meets Expectations	Does Not Meet Expectations
urgency) with availability of clinical service (provider office, urgent care, ED, etc.).						
6.12. Provides care advice to caller specific to their needs.						
6.13. Evaluates and documents the caller's understanding of recommended advice.						
6.14. Evaluates and documents the caller's intended action.						
6.15. Closes call by allowing caller to express resolution of expressed needs and/or additional needs/concerns.						
6.16. Schedules call back for caller as defined by need and/or policy.						
7. Documents caller encounters in the system that are:						
7.1. Entered concurrently with encounter.						
7.2. Uses appropriate and correctly spelled medical terminology.						
7.3. Reflective of assessed needs, recommended action, understanding and intended response of caller for each interaction.						
7.4. Reflects plan of care specific to the actual or potential health needs of the caller.						

TELEHEALTH NURSING PRACTICE ORIENTATION COMPETENCIES

EMPLOYEE: _____   **HIRE DATE:** _____   **PRECEPTOR:** _____

Orientation Competencies	Novice/Expert Weight Factor	Tested	Observed	Exceeds Expectations	Meets Expectations	Does Not Meet Expectations
8. Demonstrates appropriate management and documentation of calls if computer system is down.						
9. Complies with department and organizational policies and procedures related to:						
9.1. Managing emergency medical system or crisis intervention referrals.						
9.2. Confidentiality of caller encounters.						
9.3. Safety practices required by nature of work.						
9.4. Reporting of incidents.						
9.5. Risk management procedures.						
9.6. Mandated reporting policies.						
10. Demonstrates concern for cost-effective operations by working productively to reduce inefficiencies.						
10.1. Meets attendance standards.						
10.2. Consistently reports to work on time.						
10.3. Uses time productively by coordinating tasks, avoiding excessive socialization, completing work timely, and using slow time to department advantage.						
10.4. Agrees to work flexible schedule as needed.						

Proposed compJuly.com
Carole Becker, MS, RN
07/12/99

07/08/99

TELEHEALTH NURSING PRACTICE ORIENTATION COMPETENCIES

EMPLOYEE: _____ **HIRE DATE:** _____ **PRECEPTOR:** _____

Orientation Competencies	Novice/Expert Weight Factor	Tested	Observed	Exceeds Expectations	Meets Expectations	Does Not Meet Expectations
11. Accepts personal responsibility for maintaining and improving knowledge and skills.						
11.1. Attends all required education and competency programs directly related to practice area without prompting.						
11.2. Initiates and participates in a wider variety of educational programs relevant to practice area, healthcare trends and new clinical developments.						
11.3. Requests coaching and assistance from preceptors/other experienced staff when needed.						
11.4 Assists team members as needed without prompting.						
11.5 Design and presents unit education programs based on assessed needs of staff.						
12. Actively participates in department CQI program.						
12.1. Demonstrates adaptability and supports self-directed work groups.						
12.2. Actively participates in achieving work group goals.						
12.3. Responds positively to opportunities for improving services by implementing defined action plans.						
12.4. Participates in system-wide CQI teams as assigned.						
12.5. Evaluate client case outcome.						
12.6. Identify research questions.						

Proposed compJuly.com
Carole Becker, MS, RN
07/12/99

07/08/99

TELEHEALTH NURSING PRACTICE ORIENTATION COMPETENCIES

EMPLOYEE: _____ **HIRE DATE:** _____ **PRECEPTOR:** _____

Orientation Competencies	Novice/Expert Weight Factor		Tested	Observed		Exceeds Expectations	Meets Expectations	Does Not Meet Expectations
12.7. Evaluate nursing research findings.								

RECOMMENDATIONS: _____

_____

_____

_____

_____

COMMENTS: _____

_____

_____

_____

EMPLOYEE'S SIGNATURE: _____ PRECEPTOR'S SIGNATURE: _____

DATE: _____ DATE: _____

Proposed compJuly.com
Carole Becker, MS, RN
07/12/99

07/08/99

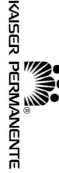

KAISER PERMANENTE ®

**Case Study for Clinical Competency
Prevention Department, Kaiser Permanente, Colorado**

Case study is one method to determine competency following orientation or education for a patient condition. Individual organizations can determine novice to expert responses for knowledge base and critical thinking. Technical skills may also be assessed when the case study is used as a mock scenario.

This Case Study was developed for the RN Lipid Management Pilot for Kaiser-Permanente, Colorado. As a collaborative effort by medicine, nursing, clinical pharmacy and dietary, it was designed to assist in determining baseline knowledge of a disease process and ability to apply the use of an algorithm in assisting the patient and health care team to manage the condition.

A healthy 55 year old white female presents for a physical examination. She has not been to a doctor in ten years and states that she has been healthy. Family history reveals that her father died of heart attack at age 55. Her brother had a heart attack at age 44. Her age is 76, and she has a history of hypertension. The patient has no history of tobacco use, although her husband smokes in the house. Her diet consists of fast food once weekly, otherwise she cooks at home, frequently frying foods in Crisco. Her activity includes a weekly walk around the park but is limited because of bilateral leg cramping with activity. She is on no prescription medication. There are no prior lipid panels available for review. B/P is 155/94, height 66 inches, weight 150, BMI 24.

Following her examination a fasting lipid panel is ordered. The results are:

Total cholesterol	280
Triglycerides	130
HDL	30
LDL	189
LDL/HDL ratio	5.4
FBS	108
TSH	4.8

<u>Questions</u>

1. What are her non-lipid and CAD equivalent risk factors? What are other considerations re: lifestyle or environment for the patient management?

2. Identify her risk level for CAD and record her LDL cholesterol goal (using the Primary Care R.N. Lipid Guideline)?

3. Identify important areas that relate to Therapeutic Lifestyle Counseling for this patient? How might you counsel this patient to help her prioritize behavior changes to focus on?

4. What are your recommendations to this patient to help her achieve reduction in her LDL cholesterol level? When should she repeat cholesterol testing?

189

Ambulatory Care Nursing Orientation and Competency
B-5: Clincial Nurse Study

The following fasting lipid profile is received 12 weeks later. The patient has followed your previous recommendations: no longer using Crisco for cooking, weight loss of 5 pounds, and increased walking to ten minutes twice daily. Her chart shows documentation that she attended cholesterol class. FLP results follow:

Total cholesterol	202
Triglycerides	140
HDL	38
LDL	136
LDL/HDL ratio	3.6
ALT	29

5. What are your recommendations to her now and when should she have her next fasting lipid profile? Do you need to order any other lab tests prior to implementing recommendations per guidelines?

The patient's FLP seven weeks later follow:

Total cholesterol	180
Triglycerides	145
HDL	38
LDL	113
LDL/HDL ratio	3.0
ALT	30
Cr	0.8

6. What are your recommendations to help achieve further cholesterol reduction to get LDL cholesterol below the goal of 100?

The patient's FLP six weeks later follow:

Total cholesterol	165
Triglycerides	132
HDL	40
LDL	98
LDL/HDL ratio	2.5
ALT	35

7. What are your final recommendations to this patient including when to check the next lipid panel?

INITIAL AND NEW COMPETENCY ASSESSMENT FORM

BUSINESS UNIT:	DEPARTMENT:

EMPLOYEE NAME (Print):	JOB TITLE:

COMPETENCY STATEMENT	Staff member will be able to operate the Laerdal Suction Unit

A. REASONS FOR SELECTION	☐ ≠ Risk, ≠ volume ☐ Regulatory Requirements/Mandate ☒ Safety Issue ☐ Performance Issue
	☒ ≠ Risk, ↓ volume ☐ P.I. Data ☐ IC Finding ☐ Other (Identify)

B. REFERENCES	☐ Performance Checklist ☐ Standards of Care Manual ☐ Policy & Procedure Manual
	☐ Other (Identify)

C. BEHAVIORAL CRITERIA	D. DIMENSIONS C - Critical Thinking I - Interpersonal Skills T - Technical Skills	E. ASSESSMENT				F. VALIDATION METHODS 1. Direct observation (actual/simulated) 2. Indirect observation (reported by peers, others) 3. Documented results of written test 4. Documented skills/ competency checklist involving techniques, procedures, etc. 5. Attendance/participation record at meetings, training, and education programs 6. Patient's commendations both positive and negative 7. Medical record review reflective of quality and accuracy of documentatic 8. Other: Specify -
		Date	Initials	Date	Initials	
Attach vacuum inlet connector tubing to vacuum inlet	T					1
Attach patient suction tubing to patient inlet	T					1
Turn on by turning operating knob to required suction setting	T					1
Attach Yankaeur suction device to patient suction tubing	T					1
Suction patient	T					1

INITIAL AND NEW COMPETENCY ASSESSMENT FORM (continued)

Empty suction canister and replace with a new canister	T					1

G. If any of the behavioral criteria cannot be validated, document the reason and corrective action below:

H. Validators:

INITIALS	PRINT NAME / TITLE	INITIALS	PRINT NAME / TITLE

Employee Name: _____ **Signature:** _____ **Date:** _____

Dept. Head/Manager: _____ **Signature:** _____ **Date:** _____

Reprinted with permission from North Shore Long Island Jewish Health System.

Safety Measures: Medication/Immunization Preparation, Administration, and Documentation

Goal: To safely prepare, administer, and document completion of a medication order.

STEPS	PURPOSE/RATIONALE	DATE	INITIALS	COMMENTS
EQUIPMENT AND SUPPLIES	Have all equipment available to be successful			
Written MD order (drug name, strength, dose, and route of administration				
PDR/Medication Binder	Gather resources needed if unfamiliar with product			
The medication/immunization container				
Correct equipment for dispensing/ administration				
Patient Record	Must document			
PROCEDURAL STEPS				
1. Read the order and clarify any questions with the MD.	To reduce error by confirming and clarifying			
2. Familiarize yourself with the product. If you are unfamiliar with the medication/ immunization, refer to the PDR, Medication Binder, and product insert.	Always know what you are giving BEFORE giving. Determine the purpose of the medication/ immunization, common side effects, typical dose, and any pertinent precautions or contraindications.			
3. When a clinic medication is being replaced with something similar, yet has a different name and/or is from a different manufacturer, consider the medication to be "New" and one you are not familiar with.	Similar medications or vaccines/immunizations that have a different name or come from a different manufacturer need to be treated as "Unfamiliar" and therefore staff need to read the product insert to confirm proper preparation and administration.			

4. Use the "7 Rights": • Right patient • Right drug • Right dose • Right route • Right time • Right technique • Right documentation	Risk reduction by reducing the possibility of a medication error			
5. In a well-lit and quiet medication room, with the MD order in hand, compare the product with the order and confirm right medication.	To avoid distraction and possible error			
6. Based on the information on the product label and the dose ordered by the MD, perform calculations needed to match MD order. Confirm with MD.	Confirm "Right dose"			
7. Wash your hands.	Infection control			
8. Compare the written order with the label on the vial when you remove it from storage. Check the expiration date on the container and dispose of the medication if it has expired. For multiuse vials, make sure the opened date is on the vial and discard if outdated.	This is the first of 3 medication checks. Confirm "Right Drug" and make sure medication/vaccine has not expired. Follow proper use of multidose vials competency.			

9.	Compare the order with the label on the vial/ampule just before drawing it up in to the appropriate syringe. Make certain that the strength on the label matches the order or that you dispense the correctly calculated dose.	This is the second of 3 medication checks. Refer to injection competency for needle choice.			
10.	Dispense the medication according to sterile technique/ clinic standards/infection control standards.	Refer to the Medication Binder in the medication room. Adhere to standards to assure safe preparation of medication.			
11.	**Along with a coworker**, compare the label and expiration date and confirm accurate preparation of medication/ vaccine/immunization and the MD order before returning the vial to storage/disposal.	This is the third of 3 medication checks.			
12.	Introduce yourself to the patient; verbally identify the patient by his or her name using the printed order sheet.	Identification of the patient prevents errors, and explanations are a means of gaining implied consent and patient cooperation. Using the order sheet allows for the patient to look and confirm name and provides a tool to use to make notes for later documentation in Epic.			
13.	Explain the procedure to the patient including the name of the medication/immunization and why it is being given. Determine/confirm any allergies the patient may have prior to administration.	To educate the patient about the medication/immunization along with allergy verification			

14.	Wash your hands.	Infection control			
15.	Administer medication/ immunization using appropriate equipment for administration along with proper site choice and preparation according to acceptable infection control practices and clinic standards.	Need for particular equipment Use Medication Binder as resource to determine appropriate anatomical site and equipment (size needle/syringe) for administration of medication.			
16.	Educate the patient on the purpose of the medication/ immunization and common side effects. For injections, remind patient to monitor site for any signs of irritation and/or infection.	Patients need to know what the MD ordered and what to look out for regarding side effects.			
17.	Instruct patient to wait for 20-30 minutes after administration as a precaution against a possible allergic reaction.	Monitor the patient for any side effects or allergic reactions and let the MD know if any occur and document appropriately.			
18.	Release the right order and document in patient chart medication/immunization given, site, and patient response. For immunizations, do not forget to document lot numbers, expiration dates, and VIS sheet given to patient.				

Young, A.P., & Proctor, D.B. (2007). Vital signs. In *The medical assistant: An applied learning approach* (10th ed., pp. 682). St. Louis, MO: Saunders.

Instrument Cleaning, Wrapping/Packaging, and Sterilization Competency

Pre-Cleaning:

1. Applies appropriate PPE – eyewear and mask or face shield, impervious long sleeve gown, and gloves

2. Immerse instruments in approved enzymatic cleaner per manufacturer's directions.

3. Discards precleaning solution after use.

Cleaning:

1. Washes hands.

2. Applies personal protective equipment (PPE) – eyewear and mask or face shield, impervious long sleeve gown, and gloves.

3. Pre-rinses instruments under cold running water to remove any visible soil.

4. Drains basket or utilizes mechanical device to lift out individual instruments.

5. Places instruments in appropriate container with manufacturer approved enzymatic detergent.
   - Leaves hinged instruments in open position and disassembles those with removable parts.
   - Labels basin with product name and date mixed. (Secondary label per EHS Hazardous Communication Policy.)
   - Instruments are soaked per manufacturer's guidelines.

6. Scrubs all surfaces with scrub brush, pipe cleaners, or other cleaning tools, paying special attention to serrated edges, box locks, and other hard to reach places.
   - Must be scrubbed while submerged in enzymatic cleaner to prevent aerosolization of BBP.
   - Brushes and cleaning tools are replaced when needed.
   - No metal brushes are used.
   - Discards enzymatic detergent after use.

7. Rinses instruments thoroughly in cool tap water.

8. If Ultrasonic machine is used:
   - Runs cycle per manufacturer's recommendations.
   - Removes instruments from pan when cycle complete and rinses in tap or distilled water per manufacturer's guidelines.
   - Allows to air dry completely. Towels, etc. will leave lint.

Milking of Instruments:

1. After cleaning, places hinged instruments and those with movable parts in a milk solution (prepared per Manufacturer's guidelines).

2. If new solution, marks container with contents, date of preparation, expiration date (**14 days post preparation**) and initials. (Secondary label per EHS Hazardous Communication Policy.) Discards if solution has separated, has gray tint, or has reached expiration date. **Soaking bin should be washed and disinfected between each preparation.**

3. Immerses instruments briefly in the milk solution per manufacturer's guidelines.

4. Removes (**DO NOT RINSE**) and allows to air dry.

Inspection:

1. Checks instruments for the following prior to packaging:
   - Hinged instruments for ease of opening and alignment of jaws and teeth.
   - Sharp or semi-sharp instruments for sharpness.
   - All instruments for cracks, chips, sharp edges, or worn spots.
   - Malleable instruments for dents and bends.

2. Removes from service **ANY** instruments with any defects and turns into to appropriate person for repair.

Instrument Cleaning, Wrapping/Packaging, and Sterilization Competency

Packaging for Sterilization:

1.	Heavier instruments are always inserted or placed in the wrap first.		
2.	Curved tips are always pointed in the same direction.		
3.	Sharp tips can be covered with gauze or special tip covers for protection.		
4.	Cupped or concave instruments are positioned to avoid water/condensation collection.		

Wrapping:

1.	Uses only the one-step wrap in appropriate size for contents. **DO NOT CUT WRAP TO SIZE.**		
2.	Places the steam indicator in the center of pack. One end should be visible when pack opened.		
3.	All instruments must be in the open position or disassembled to their smallest parts.		
4.	Separates the metal bowls/basins with appropriate material (e.g., gauze, towel) to prevent condensation and expose all surfaces to sterilization.		
5.	Secures with a MAXIMUM of 3 strips of appropriate steam indicator tape.		
6.	Labels the package using a special waterproof pen: ∨ Date of sterilization ∨ Load # ∨ Initials of person preparing package		

Peel Pack/Pouch:

1.	Selects appropriate size package.		
2.	Places the steam indicator in package so it is visible from outside the pack/pouch.		
3.	All instruments must be in the open position or disassembled to their smallest parts.		
4.	Protects sharp points with gauze or tip protectors.		
5.	Seals open end of package ensuring even seal without wrinkles and excessive air. Air acts as a barrier to heat and steam.		
6.	Labels the package using a special waterproof pen: ∨ Date of sterilization ∨ Load # ∨ Initials of person preparing package		

Autoclave:

1.	Ensures weekly biological monitor result is on file and logged.		
2.	Describes proper procedure for Biological Monitoring referring to package directions.		
3.	Describes the proper procedure for a positive result.		
4.	Completes autoclave log each time autoclave is run, monitor is sent, or maintenance is performed.		
5.	Follows Manufacturer's directions for the loading and operation of the autoclave ensuring that packs are loaded in a manner that allows for free steam and air circulation.		
6.	Places all pouches in the same direction.		
7.	Sets autoclave controls for the appropriate type of packaging.		
8.	Does not **EVER** use the "Unwrapped or Flash" cycles.		

Instrument Cleaning, Wrapping/Packaging, and Sterilization Competency

9. Articulates reasons for instrument recall/resterilization and makes appropriate notation on log:
   - Failed biological monitor
   - Visible condensation – repackages and resterilizes single package if only one; repackages and resterilizes entire load if more than 1 package affected.
   A PACKAGE WITH CONDENSATION MUST NEVER BE USED
   - Steam indicators have not changed to appropriate color
   - Package integrity concerns; compromised storage and handling conditions

10. Verifies knowledge and performance of routine maintenance per manufacturer's recommendations.

11. Has appropriate autoclave cleaner and maintenance supplies available (list):
    - ➤ Distilled water
    - ➤ Autoclave cleaner
    - ➤ Others(s) _____

Comments:

Appendix C

Professional Practice

Ambulatory Care Nursing Orientation and Competency
C-1 Medical Record Review Tool

KELSEY-SEYBOLD CLINIC - QUALITY MANAGEMENT
NURSING STAFF MEDICAL RECORD REVIEW

Name _____
Site _____
Review Date: _____

Employee Number _____
Dept _____
Reviewer: _____

Chart no.	DOB	Chart no.	DOB
1		4	
2		5	
3			

	#1	#2	#3	#4	#5	Actual	Possible
1. Direct Patient Care: Rooms patient, gathers information							
Pediatric Specific							
1. FOC: Measured and graphed birth to 12 month							
2. BP: Annually (3-6 years), every 2 years (6-18 years)							
3. Growth Chart: Ht and Wt current to age							
4. Immunization Record Documentation: Immunizations documented appropriately, i.e., authorization, date, dose, mfg, lot #, site, signature							
5. TB screen completed annually age 1-18 yr.							
6. Lead screen completed at 9 – 12 mos. and at 2 yr.							
7. Other tests: Peak flow, urine dip, hemocult, pregnancy, finger stick glucose, documented correctly							
Adult Specific							
1. Adult: Weight, Height, Vital Signs							
2. Advanced Directive: given opportunity for info, forms							
3. Adult immunizations: Tetanus q 10 yr.							
4. Pneumovax (age 65)							
5. Other tests: Peak flow, urine dip, hemocult, pregnancy, finger stick glucose, documented correctly							
OB Specific							
1. LMP							
2. Last PAP date							
3. Last Mammogram date							
Management of Information							
1. Encounter record identified with patient name and MR#							
2. Clinical Profile: Allergy/Adverse Reaction or NKA documented current to this visit							
3. Clinical Profile: Medication List current to this visit							
4. Entries authenticated (signed) with legal, legible signature and credentials							
5. Management of patient information (MOPI) audit in compliance							
6. Test results communicated within guidelines (2 weeks)							
Education of Patient & Family							
1. Educational needs documented (education sheet) and updated							
2. Educational materials (brochures, sheets, booklets) given to patient documented							
3. Learning preference documented (ie language preference, verbal, hands on)							
Pain Specific							
1. Pain documented Level (0-5)							
Legibility of Documentation							
TOTALS							

Cleveland Clinic Nurse On Call - Nursing Skills Assessment
Phone Interaction / Sharp Focus Documentation

	Call Time:			Call Time:			Call Time:			Call Time:		
	Yes	No	N/A	Yes	No	N/A	Yes	No	N/A	Yes	No	N/A
GREETING												
Greets caller couteously												
Utilizes proper opening script (identifies self, services, RN, recorded line)												
Assesses appropriateness of NOC for the caller's concern												
Accurately classifies type of call (SBC, Health Info, Physician Referral)												
Gathers appropriate demographic data												
Comments:												
PROTOCOL UTILIZATION												
Quickly indentifies priority signs / symptoms												
Selects appropriate protocol (overrides)												
Gathers & documents appropriate medical and symptom history (age, allergies, medications, etc)												
Assess pain on 1/10 scale and current method of pain control. Documents in Sharp Focus												
Upgrades recommendation as needed (Confused Adult, Foreign Speaking)												
Makes recommendation / referral per specific protocol												
Offers meds recommendation per protocol												
Offers & documents interim care measures												
Evaluate understanding of recommendation via caller feedback												
Nurse notes reflect care / recommendations provided												
Comments:												
HEALTH INFORMATION/EDUCATION												
Provides accurate and thorough information												
Verbally states source of all information												

HEALTH INFORMATION/EDUCATION - continued													
Refers to appropriate resources for addition information or support													
Requests permission to send additional or printed information													
Comments:													
PHYSICIAN REFERRAL													
Offers and documents referral service													
Selects appropriate specialty													
Identifies specific criteria necessary for referral (location, insurance)													
Transfers caller to appropriate department and acts as liason when needed													
Documents referral accurately													
Comments:													
COMMUNICATION SKILLS													
Conveys a positive image of organization													
Maintains a courteous, calm, professional demeanor													
Exhibits ability to adapt to different personalities and emotions													
Assumes control of call, listens attentively, interjects appropriately and elicts necessary information													
Takes time with caller when appropriate; efficient without compromising quality													
Uses simple, direct language caller understands													
Does not interrupt nor interjects for caller													
Speaks at a moderate rate with expressive modulation of tone													
Maintains controll of call													
Does not eat, drink, chew gum or conduct other activities which interfere with conversation													

205

Comments:												
CLOSING SPEECH												
Ends call efficiently												
Offers instructions to call back or seek medical care if condition worsens, new symptoms or concern regarding condition												
Reviews recommendations and requests feedback to evaluate caller understanding												
Disconnects last												
Comments:												

Name of Operator:_____

Name of Reviewer:_____

Date of Review:_____

Reprinted with permission from the Cleveland Clinic Foundation

RN Triage Refresher Training (Didactic) Part I
August 9, 2008

1. **Goals for RN Triage**
   The RN will:
   A. Determine the patient acuity: triages care prioritization according to patient complaint, injury, and illness of patients over the entire age spectrum (pediatrics through geriatrics), utilizing the 5 tiered patient classification system and rapid assessment of physical, developmental, and psychological need; assign an appropriate acuity level (Emergency Nursing Association [ENA]).
   B. *Organizational Goal for RN Triage (PMG)* – "To improve the service provided to the Urgent Care patient by improving the cycle time for a visit and improving the quality of the visit." In clinical practice, the role of RN triage nurse is to quickly assess (in less than 5 minutes) the patient, make a triage decision, and transfer to the appropriate setting (Urgent Care or Emergency Room).

2. **Triage Nurse Qualifications** (Excerpt from Sheehy, *Textbook of Emergency Nursing*, 5th ed.)

3. **RN Triage References:**
   A. "Triage Protocol," Presbyterian Emergency Services (HPP)
   B. Emergency Severity Index (ESI): Chapter 3 – Introduction to the Emergency Severity Index
   C. Excerpt on "ED Nursing Practice in Action" from *Emergency Nursing Malpractice* by Patricia Iyer (p. 635)
   D. Standing Orders (3) in Urgent Care Clinics
   E. Provider Consultations for special situations

4. **Emergency Severity Index, Version 4:** (Agency for Healthcare Quality & Research)
   A. An Overview of the ESI, Version 4 Algorithm (DvD)
   B. ESI Level 2 (Chapter 4)
   C. Expected Resource Needs (Chapter 5)
   D. The Role of Vital Signs in Triage (Chapter 6)
   E. Case Scenario Discussion (30 cases)

5. **Triage Documentation** – Nursing Intake/Assessment form for PMG Urgent Care Clinics
   A. Critical assessment areas for RN liability (see Nursing Intake form)
   B. Patient Hand-off Process to:
      I. Urgent Care Clinic – Triage Category 2 (immediate intervention), Category 3 (urgent)
      II. Emergency Department
         a. Required chart documentation and advanced ER communications
         b. PMG Transfer Policy (Draft), from RN Triage and from UC to ED

6. **Competency Elements** – Complete prior to Part 2 Class (scheduled in 6-8 weeks)
   A. Clinical observation – At least 4 hours or greater with any Urgent Care RN
   B. Clinical observation with Rio Rancho ED Triage RN (4 hours) (RRUC only)
   C. Perform RN Triage on at least 3 shifts utilizing the ESI algorithm and meet the documentation requirements for RN Triage (for audit purposes)
   D. By December 31, 2008, complete the 2008 RN Triage Review in HPP
   E. To obtain a copy of *ESI Implementation Handbook*, Version 4, call 1-800-358-9295 (AHRQ) and request Publication 305-0046-2 (free of charge)

7. **Course Evaluation**

RN Triage Training Part 2
November 21, 2008

Purpose of class: Complete review of the ESI case scenarios and discuss lessons learned from triage observation and supervision with colleagues. Results from a retrospective review of triage documentation will provide an opportunity for improvement in triage assessment.

I. Triage Experiences with Preceptors   45 MIN

    A. Take-away points? Changes in practice?

    B. Scheduled time with ED Triage RN?

    C. "Red Flags in Urgent Care Documentation" (see *Nursing Malpractice* by Patricia Iyer)

II. Triage Decisions   90 MIN

    A. Review ESI Triage Algorithm, v.4 (poster)

    B. Discuss patient assessment in light of resources needed and abnormal vital signs on the triage decision

    C. RN Triage Documentation Audit

    D. Case Scenarios (Vital Signs)

III. Nursing Standards & Regulatory Requirements   60 MIN

    A. "Organizational/Systems Role of the Ambulatory Care Nurse," Chapter 2, *A Guide to Ambulatory Care Nursing Orientation & Competency Assessment* (AAACN, 2005) (hand-outs provided)

        1. Dimension 7: Priority/Management and Supervision

        2. Dimension 13: Legal Issues: (Consent, Transfers, Abandonment, Reportable Situations, Documentation, Tele-Health, Regulation of Nursing Practice)

    B. NM Nurse Practice Act (Rules 16.12.1.1 – 16.12.1.8) – Patient Abandonment Rule Relationship with RN hand-off to ED RN

V. Continuing Nursing Education for Urgent Care Practice   15 MIN

    A. www.pearls.com - see Ambulatory Nursing Topics (Presbyterian Foundation Gift)

    B. Urgent Care Clinic Continuing Education Program

    C. *Nursing Spectrum Magazine* (free) monthly CNE topics

    D. Perry & Potter's *Textbook of Medical Surgical Nursing*

    E. Sheehy's *Textbook of Emergency Nursing*

VI. Course Evaluation   10 MIN

References

Gilboy, N., Tanabe, P., Travers, D.A., Rosenau, A.M., & Eitel, D.R. (2005) *Emergency severity index, version 4: Implementation handbook.* AHRQ Publication No. 05-0046-2. Rockville, MD: Agency for Healthcare Research & Quality.

Iyer, P.W., & Levin, B.J. (Eds.). (2007). *Nursing malpractice* (3rd ed.). Tucson, AZ: Lawyers & Judges Publishing Company, Inc.

Newberry, L. (2003). *Sheehy's emergency nursing: Principles and practice* (5th ed.). St. Louis, MO: Mosby Elsevier.

Created by Joan M. Pate, MS, RN, PMG Urgent Care Clinic, Rio Rancho, New Mexico.

Ambulatory Care Nursing Orientation and Competency
C-4: RN Triage Training Part 2

Appendix D

Orientation Plan Examples

University of Michigan Health System
Ambulatory Care Services
RN Orientation

Day 1 (w/ACS ENC)	Introduction/ needs assessment	Review of Orientation Plan	Ambulatory Nursing Overview (AAACN/Digiscript) Organizational structure - (broad)	Discussion: Differences in AC Nursing vs. other specialties	Education resources	Computer module
Day 2 (unit-level)	Preceptor introduction(s), learning styles, review of needs assessment/ orientation plan	Tour of unit/workspace, staff introductions, organizational structure - (unit), unit resources	Clinic operations (opening, closing, administrative policies/procedures), shadowing w/ preceptor	Skills checklist, review of orientation competencies	Communications (telephone, voice-mail, e-mail, verbal, written, fax, confidentiality), Documentation	Safety/Emergency including AED competency
Day 3 (w/ ACS ENC)	Role clarification, Q&A, assessment of preceptor "fit"	Clinical Practice – Triage and Assessment, Technical Skills and Clinical Practice – (selected content) (AAACN/Digiscript)	Communications: Interpersonal Skills/Cultural Competency, Telephone/Multimedia, Documentation (AAACN/Digiscript)	Telephone Nursing Practice Administration and Practice Standards (AAACN)	Telephone Triage video (Mosby), UMHS Telephone Nursing Practice competency	UMHS Patient Education resources/practices
Day 4 (unit-level)	Shadowing w/ preceptor	Clinic paperwork, protocols, delegation guidelines, other written guidelines, Advance Directives, coordination of care	Use of dual headsets for Telephone Nursing Practice	Focus on unit-specific skills	Con't. shadowing	Con't. shadowing
Day 5 (w/ACS ENC)	Legal and Regulatory Issues, Systems – Operations and Fiscal Management (AAACN/Digiscript), Core Curriculum pp. 64-67, 84-95, 110-123	Delegation module	Assessment/Re-assessment guidelines, billing for nursing services, prior authorization process(es)	Prescription refill process	Review of relevant job descriptions (i.e. MA, LPN, CNI/CNII/CNIII, etc.)	Quality Improvement and JCAHO modlues
Day 6 (unit-level)	Skills "lab"	Skills "lab" con't.	Time with clerical staff as appropriate (i.e. scheduling appts. included in role)	Preceptor observation of orientee's delivery of age-appropriate care	JCAHO "walk through" or discussion w/ Nurse Manager	Review of unit Quality Improvement initiative

211

University of Michigan Health System
Ambulatory Care Services
RN Orientation

Day 7 (w/ ACS ENC)	Issues and Trends – Professional Roles, Care Management/Disease Management, Client Education (AAACN/Digiscript)	Clinical Practice (Core Curriculum – population specific content)	Explore UMHS Continuing Care Services Website(s)	Navigate UMHS Policies/Procedures	Problem-based learning scenario	Completion of mandatory competencies as needed
Day 8 (unit-level)	Shadow LPN	Shadow MA	Primary Care track – Allergy Clinic experience (experience varies w/ track)	Allergy Clinc con't	Allergy Clinic con't.	Allergy Clinic con't.
Day 9 (w/ ACS ENC)	Tracks con't	Tracks con't	Tracks con't.	Tracks con't	Tracks con't.	Tracks con't.
Day 10 (unit-level)	Work independently w/ preceptor as back-up	Work independently w/ preceptor as back-up	Determine unmet learning needs	Define plan for meeting unmet learning needs	Identification of post-orientation resources	Completion of evaluations

Reprinted with permission from Candia B. Laughlin and the University of Michigan

UNIVERSITY OF COLORADO HOSPITAL

AMBULATORY CARE TEAM CHARGE NURSE ORIENTATION RECORD

Name: _____ Date: _____

Unit: _____ Manager/Director: _____

Instructions   Manager/Director: Please send original white copy to Human Resources for the employee's UCH personnel file. Place yellow copy in employee's department personnel file.

UCH Clinical Orientation

- Welcome
- Patient Education
- Patient Comfort and Safety
- Team Communications
- Nursing Philosophy and Role
- Risk Management
- UEXCEL

- Medication Delivery Systems
- Skin Assessment
- Hospital Tour and Library Orientation
- Sedation
- Pain Assessment
- Changing Patient Condition

ACES Orientation

- Introduction to ACES
- Introduction to Insurance/Managed Care
- Introduction to CICP/Medicare etc.
- Role of the Nurse in Ambulatory
- Interpreter Services
- Clinical skills: telephone triage, venipuncture, Intravenous, Immunizations, glucometer

- Medical Records and Patient Rights
- Telephone and Telephone etiquette
- Clinical Emergencies
- Intranet skills (CWS)
- Charge Nurse Role
- Changing Patient Condition

Signature (Director / Manager / Educator / Designee)   Title   Date

---

To be completed within two years post hire.
Course offered through UCH Human Resources and Professional Resources

- Evidenced Based Practice
- Preceptor Training
- Managing Diversity
- Management Development Series-session 2

- Policies and Procedures
- Examining Conflict

The above was reviewed and incorporated into the employees professional development plan

Signature (Director / Manager / Educator / Designee)   Title   Date

---

Unit / Division Orientation

- Charge Nurse Clinical Orientation
- Clinical Nurse Orientation Checklist

_____ has completed all required components of orientation.

Signature (Director / Manager / Educator / Designee)   Title   Date

General Orientation Schedule Outline

For

Cleveland Clinic Nurse on Call Telehealth Nursing Practice Program

Purpose: To provide a comprehensive orientation to the operation of Nurse on Call. The process is established and monitored by the NOC trainer and supported by selected mentors. Each nurse is provided an orientation manual, select reading materials, and an orientation schedule and checklist. The process includes practice sessions, listening to calls with mentor, taking calls with mentor and continuous feedback. The orientation period is 4-6 weeks

I. Introduction and overview of CCF Nurse on Call
A. Introduction to staff and tour of department
B. Meet with Call Center Manager
   1 Organization of department and job descriptions
C. Meet with Senior RN to review staffing / hours procedures
D. Meet with Director of RHA
   1 Division / Department organizational chart
E. Functions and review of NOC program
   1. Selected readings assigned

11. Scope of Service
A. Community Callers
   1. Health Information
   2. Symptom based triage
   3. Physician / Service Referral
B. Cleveland Clinic Established Patient Callers - After Hrs Management
   1. FHCs
   2. GIM & Pediatrics
   3. Sub-speciality practices
C. On-Call physician schedules
D. Relationship / interaction with Appointment Center Schedulers

IV. Standard Operating Procedures
A. Orientation to phone system
   1. Skill based call routing and reporting
   2. Recording of calls / Confidentiality of calls
   3. Transfer / Conference Calls
B. Call Centre Approved Reference Resources
   1. NOC references
   2. CCF Department references
   3. Community Resources

C. Standardized Forms
  1. Encounter Forms
  2. Physician referral letters
  3. Health Information letters
  4. Sports Health Letter
  5. Special Call Reports

V. Symptom - based calls

A. NOC Call Process
  1. Classifying the call
  2. Priority Evaluation
  3. Collecting Demographics
  4. Protocol Selection
    a. Overrides/Silent red flags
    b. Past history
  5. Assessment
    a. Scholar
    b. Child
      1. Level of activity
      2. Level of hydration
  6. Recommendations
    a. Emergent
    b. 24 Hour
    c. 72 Hour
    d. Interim care
    e. Caller understanding
  7. Closing Statement

B. Documentation
  1. Open Ended Questions (Scholar)
  2. Directed Questions
  3. Nursing Assessment of Collected Data
  4. Recommendation
  5. Patients Plan of Action
  6. Special Call Report Forms

C. Specialized Programs and Protocols
  1. Asthma Disease Management
  2. CHF Disease Management
  3. Seizure Disease Management
  4. Sports Health Calls

5. WalMart Health information Line
6. Med Well Line
5. EpiCare
V1. Technical skills Training
A. Preceptor Supervision
B. Independent Skills Assessment
C. Evaluation

NEW EMPLOYEE ORIENTATION SCHEDULE FOR RN, LVN, MA & OA

Employee Name: _____

Mgr or Preceptor: _____   Location: _____

	Day / Location	Morning	Afternoon
E L L A	**MONDAY - Week 1** Date: ___/___/___ Administrative Business Center (8900 Lakes at 610 Drive)	**Morning, 8:00-11:45, Room 11** Registration and check-in Introductions/Logistics/Schedules Company History & Organization Vision, Mission, Values Customer Service Standards ***Lunch & ID badges***	**Afternoon, 12:45-5:00, Room 11** NEO Manual and Packet Safety and Health Activities Benefits Overview Reminders, Dismissal
E M P L O Y E E S	**TUESDAY - Week 1** Date: ___/___/___ Administrative Business Center (8900 Lakes at 610 Drive)	**Morning, 8:00-12:00, Room 11** Review of Vision, Mission, Values Payday Schedule, KRONOS Rewards & Recognition Program Managed Health Care Integrity Training Risk Management / Medical Records Evaluations	**Afternoon, 1:00-5:00, Rooms 25 & 26** Technical Systems Overview Intranet Telephone usage IDX Benefits Q & A
N U R S E	**WEDNESDAY - Week 1** Date: ___/___/___ Administrative Business Center (8900 Lakes at 610 Drive)	**Morning, 8:00-12:00, Room 25** Appointment setting class	**Afternoon, 1:00-5:00, Call Center** Appointment practice
O R I E N T A T I O N	**THURSDAY - Week 1** Date: ___/___/___ Administrative Business Center (8900 Lakes at 610 Drive)	**Morning, 8:00-12:00, Room 25** Chart Tracking computer class	**Afternoon, 12:30-5:00, Room 12** CPR recert if needed **1:00-5:00, Call Center** Practice making appointments in Call Center
	FRIDAY - Week 1 Date: ___/___/___ Administrative Business Center (8900 Lakes at 610 Drive)	**Morning, 8:00-12:00, Room 12** Nursing Orientation General Guidelines Rooming & Charting IDX RAD	**Afternoon, 1:00-5:00, Room 12** Forms Documentation test Managed Care and test
	MONDAY-WEEK 2 DATE: ___/___/___ Administrative Business Center (8900 Lakes at 610 Drive)	**Morning, 8:00-12:00 Room 12** Nursing Orientation cont. Lab/LabCorp access Waived testing and tests Code Blue and test	**Afternoon, 1:00-5:00pm** Telephone Standards and tests Medications and Immunizations

NEW EMPLOYEE ORIENTATION SCHEDULE FOR RN, LVN, MA & OA (continued)

	Morning 8:00-12:00 PM Room 24	Afternoon 1:00 - 5-00PM Room 24
TUESDAY -WEEK 2 **DATE:** ___/___/___ *Administrative Business Center* *(8900 Lakes at 610 Drive)*	Skills Assessment	Skills assessment cont.
WEDNESDAY - WEEK 2 **DATE:** ___/___/___ *Administrative Business Center* *(8900 Lakes at 610 Drive)*	*Morning 8:00 - 12:00 PM Room 24* Skills Assessment cont.	*Afternoon 1:00 - 5:00 PM Room 24* Skills Assessment cont.
Thurs & Fri - Week 2	**Regular Hours as scheduled at your site** Work with mentor/preceptor to complete check off list and orientation to your site	
MON - FRI, WEEKS 3, 4, 5 & 6	**Regular hours as scheduled at your site** Work with mentor/preceptor to complete check off list and orientation to your site	

Dress Code: Business casual clothes may be worn for Orientation classes at ABC

NURSES: Wear your work uniform on the last day of skills. If you complete your skills assessment on Tuesday, you will proceed to your assigned clinic. Otherwise, you will complete your skills on Wednesday.

Following the first 8 days of employment:
Triage nurses will be scheduled to attend the Telephone Triage Class
Immunization nurses will be scheduled for 3 days of Allergy injection training at Main Campus-4 in Allergy
Immunization nurses will be scheduled for 2 days of Foreign travel training.
Immunization nurses will be scheduled for Immunization Class

Reprinted with permission from the Kelsey-Seybold Clinic

218

Appendix E

Orientation Competency Validation Checklists

KELSEY-SEYBOLD CLINIC
STAFF DEVELOPMENT
COMPETENCY BASED ORIENTATION VALIDATION FORM

Name: _____RN, LVN, MA   Date: _____

Employee Number_____ ☐ Initial skills ☐ Annual skills

Performance criteria **Ear Lavage**	Validation of performance	Self assessment				Date competency met. Validators signature.	Learning options	Action plan Comments
		Have you ever done this before?		Are you competent performing?				
		NO	YES	NO	YES			
Prepare solution for irrigation temp100-105 degrees								
Explain procedure to patient								
Wears gloves. View affected ear with otoscope to see where cerumen is located								
Positions patient and places basin under ear for patient to hold to catch solution. Places towel on patient's shoulder								
Uses syringe to irrigate ear. Flow should be directed upward and to one side.								
Tilt head to side to drain extra solution								
Observes for dizziness								
Charts procedure in detail- which ear, solution used &amt, results								
Cleans/disposes of equipment								

KELSEY-SEYBOLD CLINIC
STAFF DEVELOPMENT
COMPETENCY BASED ORIENTATION VALIDATION FORM

Name: _____RN, LVN, MA   Date: _____

Employee Number_____ ☐ Initial skills ☐ Annual skills

Performance criteria **DCA 2000+ analyzer**	Validation of performance	Self assessment				Date competency met. Validators signature.	Learning options	Action plan Comments
		Have you ever done this before?		Are you competent performing?				
		NO	YES	NO	YES			
	Can perform controls and complete log							
	Can perform finger stick and collect specimen							
	Can run test							
	Provides appropriate documentation							

University of Colorado Hospital
Far Beyond the Ordinary

A CLINIC SCAVENGER HUNT

1) - Complete the first week of orientation
2) - As you locate, place initials and date in correct column
3) - Ask other staff members to help you locate
4) - Upon completion, give to care team manager

If you can not answer, contact your care team manager or preceptor for assistance

Name: _____ **Clinic:** _____

	Initials and Date
In Our Department............	
Patient Rights	
The patient rights brochures/sign are located	
The advance directive brochures are located	
The brochures on abuse are located....	
Interpretive services can be obtained by calling	
Informed consent forms used for procedures are located	
The annual consent to treat forms we use for each patient are located....	
The annual patient self assessment forms are located....	
The Patient Privacy hotline number is...	
Our compliance hot line notice is located	
Environment of Care	
Our personal protective equipment is located	
The Hazard Communication manual/ information is located	
Fire drill and emergency preparedness records are located..	
The oxygen shut off valve for our area is located .... [note – this may be N/A in some areas]. What is the protocol?	
The fire extinguishers in our department are located	
The fire pulls/fire alarms in our department are located	
Emergency exit routes from our department are located..	
The next smoke zone, i.e. where patients would be evacuated to if there were a fire in our area	
Accidental Exposure form (for testing source after an occupational exposure) is located	
Patient Care	
Take the Step for Patient Safety flyers are located...	
Patient Education materials are located..	
Patient occurrence report forms are located	
Patients with a communicable disease are isolated in _____ location	
Original Medical Records for our patients are located ...	
Our clinic:	
Our performance improvement model is posted	
Our education bulletin board is located	
Employee belongings are kept.....	
Bathrooms for patients and staff are located	
Bathroom keys are located	
The AED is located-	
O2 tank and Ambu located-	
Tackle box/code cart located-	
Plan D for our clinic is located...	

223

CLEVELAND CLINIC FOUNDATION
Ambulatory Clinic Nursing
NURSE ON CALL
ORIENTATION CHECKLIST

Name _____

Date Initiated _____

AMBULATORY NURSING GENERAL INFORMATION

Activities	Discussed - Attended		Observed		Completed		Comments
	Date	Initial	Date	Initial	Date	Initial	
CCF Administrative							
Mission Statement							
CCF Nursing Philosophy							
Table of organization							
Job description							
Probation/Performance Evals							
Payroll/ Time & Attendance							
PTO/Vacation/Attendance Policy							
Dress Code							
Calendar of Events: Amb Nsg							
Quality Management							
Quality concepts							
CCF Nsg Structure							

AMBULATORY NURSING GENERAL INFORMATION						
Activities	**Discussed - Attended**		**Observed**		**Completed**	**Comments**
	Date	Initial	Date	Initial	Date	Initial	
Nurse On Call Special Call Report Review of Sentinel Events policy						
Educational Requirements						
*Age Specific competency review						
* B.L.S. CPR						
Ambulatory Nursing Classes Offered during Orientation						
Patient Education: approved NOC sites; documentation						
Customer Service: World Class Service; Pt Satisfaction						
Telephone Triage: concepts, tips						
Social Work: Abuse policies, *Abuse videos (elder, domestic & child)						
Pharmacy: Medication Issues, Pharmacy Resources						
Inf. Control- Preventing Occupational Exposure to Bloodborne Pathogens & TB (OASHA Infection Control Video)						

AMBULATORY NURSING GENERAL INFORMATION

Activities	Discussed - Attended		Observed		Completed		Comments
	Date	Initial	Date	Initial	Date	Initial	
Safety Information							
Occupational Injury/Illness							
Fire Box/Extinguisher/alarms							
Evacuation Route Review- fire walks							
Hazcom, especially in reference to handling Toner Cartridges, etc…							
OASHA training sheet							
Review Nurse On Call Disaster Plan							
Computer Resources							
Intranet Resources							
*EPICARE Training							
*HIPAA on-line training							

indicates self-study completion or on-line programming and is not expected to be completed in class.

AAACN Education Special Interest Group

Competency Format Example

A. Competency Statement: The Ambulatory Nurse will be competent in the safe performance of Telephone Triage

Performance Criteria (Knowledge and Skill	Reference	Date Validated	Validated by:
1. Critera			
2. Criteria			

B. Example

Competency Assessment For Telephone Triage

Name _____ Job Title _____ Unit _____

Competency	Method of Verification	Date Completed
Technical Domain: 1. Demonstrates the ability to use the phone systems including voice mail, conference calling and call back features.	Return demonstration in Telephone Class Peer Observation Observer signature _____	
Critical Thinking Domain:		
Interpersonal Domain:		

Action Plan:

As outlined by the successful completion of the above criteria, this employee is competent to perform as a _____ on date _____ Yes No

Employee Signature _____ Date _____ Supervisor
Signature _____ Date: _____

New Clinical Staff Orientation Checklist – EMR
(RN, LVN, MA, CMA, OA)

Name: _____ **Emp. No.** _____

Location _____ **Department** _____

Core information will be provided onsite by your nursing supervisor and other staff. The following should be included in the instruction at the site to assure employees become fully oriented to their new position at Kelsey-Seybold Clinic.

Supervisor/Administrators/Preceptors: Please provide the following information/training.

Training Need	Date Instructed/ Completed	Instructor Signature	Employee Signature
BASICS			
Definitions ASR, CSR, HIM tech			
Log on to EPIC EMR			
Patient flow arrive to rooming			
Where procedure manual are found			
ROOMING A PATIENT			
Ck arrival in computer			
Pre-visit summary (if used)			
Escort to room			
Build smart sets			
Enter data into EMR – Vital signs and chief complaint, validate meds, allergies, immunizations, questionnaires (TB, ADHD, LEAD, Flu, others)			
Place orders			
Nurse notes			
Patient education			
Follow-up			
Stress focus on patient not computer			
Review how to manage In-box			
Related Policies Below (not to be considered complete list)			
Patient Identification PE.20.08			
Medical Record Documentation MR.002b			
Vital Signs TX.33.97			
Pain Management TX.47.00			
Scope of Patient Care Assessment PE.01.97			
Medication Administration TX.13.97			
KEEP STATION FLOW			
Check for late arrivals			
Clean and stock rooms			
Identify patient before procedures and giving meds			
Telephone management			
Check in-basket for past due test and orders			
Assist with procedures			
UR referrals			
Do not use abbreviations			
Related Policies Below (not to be considered complete list)			
Telephone Screening And Referrals CC.05.97			
See Dangerous Abbreviations List			
Medical Record Documentation MR.002b			
Medication Administration TX.13.97			
Diagnostic Test and Follow-Up Communication PE.03.98			
Utilization Review CC.03.97			

New Clinical Staff Orientation Checklist – EMR
(RN, LVN, MA, CMA, OA)

Name:		Emp. No.	
Location		Department	

	Date Instructed/ Completed	Instructor Signature	Employee Signature
FORMS			
Time off requests			
Advanced directives			
Release of Information			
Incident reporting – Midas			
Related Policies Below (not to be considered complete list)			
Vacation Hr 4.000			
Advance Directives Pr.03.97			
Release Of Information To Patient Hi.009			
Patient Complaints Pr.02.97			
MEDICATION ADMINISTRATION – RN/LVN			
Documentation			
Review P&Ps			
Floor Stock			
Controlled substances			
Peak flow meter			
Review dosage calculations			
Documentation			
Review P&Ps			
Related Policies Below (not to be considered complete list)			
Medical Record Documentation MR.002b			
Medication Administration TX.13.97			
See Dangerous Abbreviations List			
Routine Standing Orders TX.21.97			
Training Need			
Verification for anticoag, insulin, heparin			
Sample drugs			
Pharmacy ordering			
Immunizations –VIS and documentation			
Asthma action plan			
Related Policies Below (not to be considered complete list)			
Nebulizer Treatments TX.26.97			
Minimally Invasive And Minor Procedures Tx.24.97			
Diagnostic Test and Follow-Up Communication PE.03.98			
Medication Administration TX.13.97			
Medical Record Documentation MR.002b			
WAIVED TESTING (complete -learn lesson)			
Urine dip screening			
Blood Glucose			
Controls			
Strip & control care			
Pregnancy Test			
Hemoccult			
Logs QI Testing			
Related Policies Below (not to be considered complete list)			
Blood Glucose Waived Laboratory PE.13.97			
Urine Dipstick Waived Laboratory Testing PE 12.97			
Fecal Occult Blood Waived Laboratory Test PE.15.97			

New Clinical Staff Orientation Checklist – EMR
(RN, LVN, MA, CMA, OA)

Name:		Emp. No.	
Location		Department	

OTHER SKILLS ASSESSMENT (complete I-learn lesson)			
Vital signs check			
Pediatric measurements			
OB FHT			
Sterile fields			
Location and use of PPE			
OB & GYN videos for pt education			
Related Policies Below (not to be considered complete list)			
Immunization Clinic/Allergy Clinic TX.12.97			
Common Nursing Procedures TX.05.97			
Pain Management			
Vital Signs TX.33.97			

LAB RESULTS			
TeleVox			
Lab letters			
Phone pt with results			
Document results reported			
Teach Test Results Tracking process			
Management of abnormal or Life threatening result reports from LabCorp or Radiology			
Review P& P on Results reporting			
Specimen labeling			
Related Policies Below (not to be considered complete list)			
Diagnostic Test and Follow-Up Communication PE.03.98			
Clinical Laboratory Testing PE.09.97			
Labeling In-Office Collected Specimens For Laboratory Testing PE.21.07			

ABUSE RECOGNITION AND REPORTING (complete I-learn lesson)			
Elder			
Child			
Related Policy Below (not to be considered complete list)			
Management Of Suspected Abuse And Neglect PR.14.97			

TELEPHONE SCREENING – RN/LVN (complete I-learn lesson)			
Scope of practice for triage for RN, LVN, MA			
Process for collecting data			
Documentation			
After-hours calls			
Assessing signs and symptoms			
Emergency management			
Completing a call/message			
Related Policies Below (not to be considered complete list)			
Referrals to Emergency Department CC.07.97			
Telephone Screening And Referrals CC.05.97			
Utilization Review CC.03.97			
Functional Assessment PE. 08.97			

IV SKILLS (complete I-learn lesson)			
Review procedure			
Review drip rate calculation			
How to use safety devices			

New Clinical Staff Orientation Checklist – EMR
(RN, LVN, MA, CMA, OA)

Name:	Emp. No.
Location	Department

Training Need	Date Instructed /Completed	Instructor Signature	Employee Signature
Check skills			
Related Policy Below (not to be considered complete list)			
Common Nursing Procedures TX.05.97			
CATHETERIZATION (complete I-learn lesson)			
Review procedure			
Review kit content			
Check skills			
Related Policy Below (not to be considered complete list)			
Common Nursing Procedures TX.05.97			
CODE BLUE (complete I-learn lesson)			
Please Refer To Clinical Education Website For Detailed Information			
Validate current certification of CPR, ACLS, and or PALS			
Review Emergency Procedures			
Review Standing orders			
Review P&P			
Review cart contents			
Daily check			
Monthly check			
Restocking cart			
Code team responsibilities –mock code drill			
Recording forms			
CARE AND CLEANING OF INSTRUMENTS			
Please Refer To Environmental Health & Safety Web site For Detailed Information (look in Infection Control section)			
Disposable and reusable			
MA SCOPE			
MA **cannot** take verbal orders review P&P			
MAII (can give routine immunizations and apply TB skin test but **cannot** read TB test)			
MA **cannot** work directly from a standing order			
MANAGED CARE OVERVIEW			
Differences in HMO & PPO			
UR process			
Related Policies Below (not to be considered complete list)			
Care Coordination CC.06.97			
Referrals to Emergency Department CC.07.97			
MEDICAL RECORDS			
Storage and management			
HIPAA			
Patient confidentiality			
Related Policies Below (not to be considered complete list)			
Maintenance Of Health Information HI.003			
Minimizing Inadvertent Disclosures HI.002			

New Clinical Staff Orientation Checklist – EMR
(RN, LVN, MA, CMA, OA)

Name:		Emp. No.	
Location		Department	

IMAGE CAST				
De-Identification Of Patient Information Hi.018				
Image Cast How to use				
PATIENT EDUCATION				
Location resources				
Patient learning needs assessment				
Documenting				
PEER REVIEW AND SAFE HARBOR - RN & LVN				
Review Peer Review P&P. Find on Pulse HR P&Ps				
Review form location for Peer Review and Safe Harbor				
Have Nurse Sign NPA Acknowledgment form				
SITE-SPECIFIC ITEMS				
▪				
▪				
▪				
▪				
▪				
▪				
▪				
▪				
▪				
▪				

DIRECTORATE, PRIMARY CARE

ORIENTATION COMPETENCY STATEMENTS AND PERFORMANCE CRITERIA: Patient Assessment, Education, and Care

COMPETENCY STATEMENT/ PERFORMANCE CRITERIA	SELF-ASSESS	ADDITIONAL LEARNING OPTIONS	METHOD TO MEASURE	M = Met NM = Not Met	COMMENTS
Population specific care to patients.					
1. **General** a. Demonstrates knowledge and skills necessary to meet the patient's physiologic needs. b. Demonstrates knowledge and skills necessary to meet patient's psychosocial needs. 　(1) Assesses stage of development. 　(2) Assesses responses to illness (stress, fear/anxiety, crisis, loneliness, and changes in intimacy) and intervenes appropriately. 　(3) Assesses stressors (environment, self-concept, self-esteem, body-image, powerlessness, sensory overload/deprivation) and intervenes appropriately. 　(4) Assesses and integrates patient's needs related to: family/social support, religion, and culture. c. Individualizes care based upon physical, psychosocial, and/or age-specific needs. d. Provides age appropriate patient/family education.		Review and complete self-learning module on population-specific competency prior to attending Nursing Orientation. Complete population-specific competency with Preceptor.	Successfully complete post test. Orientee completes age-specific competency and submits evaluation to DTR.		
2. **Geriatric patient (ages 65 years and older)** a. Recognizes physical changes associated with aging for all body systems including cognition and sensory alterations. b. Recognizes psychosocial changes associated with aging (mentation, support systems). c. Incorporates effects of altered pharmacologic response/polypharmacy when administering prescribed medications. d. Provides patient with a safe environment.		Review and complete self-learning module on age-specific competency prior to attending Nursing Orientation. Complete age specific competency with Preceptor.	Successfully complete post test. Orientee completes age-specific competency and submits evaluation to DTR.		☐ N/A: only adult patient population is served in this clinic.
3. **Adult Patient (18-65 years old)** a. Recognizes potential concerns regarding: • role change and conflict • finances • career • child care		Review and complete self-learning module on age-specific competency prior to attending Nursing Orientation. Complete age-specific competency with Preceptor.	Successfully complete post test. Orientee completes age-specific competency and submits evaluation to DTR.		
4. **Pediatric Patient (neonate, infant, child, and adolescent)** a. Recognizes potential concerns regarding: • body image • loss of identity		Review and complete self-learning module on age-specific competency prior to attending Nursing	Successfully complete post test. Orientee completes age-		☐ N/A: only adult patient population is served in this clinic.

◆ For individuals with prior clinic experience, orientation time frames may be adjusted; however, the minimum competencies must be demonstrated prior to completing orientation. Therefore, the individual may self-assess certain skills that are agreed upon with the clinic nurse, preceptor, charge nurse, or department head.
　◆ To **self-assess**, write either '**C**' = "competent" or '**ND**' = "needs development" in the "Self-Assess" Column.
◆ In the '**Method to Measure Competency' column**, if the number of times to perform a performance criteria is not stated, it is implied that it will be demonstrated <u>one</u> time.
◆ In the '**Met/Not Met' column** write either '**M**' = "Met" or '**NM**' = "Not Met" and the orienteer's initials. Write specific needs that remain and any other helpful information in the 'comments' column.

DIRECTORATE, PRIMARY CARE

ORIENTATION COMPETENCY STATEMENTS AND PERFORMANCE CRITERIA: **Patient Assessment, Education, and Care**

COMPETENCY STATEMENT/ PERFORMANCE CRITERIA	SELF-ASSESS	ADDITIONAL LEARNING OPTIONS	METHOD TO MEASURE	M = Met NM = Not Met	COMMENTS
• peer relations • autonomy		Orientation. Complete age-specific competency with Preceptor.	specific competency and submits evaluation to DTR.		
CARDIOVASCULAR SYSTEM					
Performs a cardiovascular assessment and integrates data to determine when a patient is at risk.					
1. Assesses patient and recognizes normal and abnormal cardiovascular findings: • skin color and temperature • capillary refill • edema • symptoms – chest pain and palpitations			Evaluator confirms assessment findings. Orientee verbalizes etiologies of abnormal findings.		
2. Determines presence and quality of pulses (radial, dorsalis pedis, posterior tibial): • strong, weak, moderate, absent			Orientee verbalizes etiologies of abnormal findings.		
3. Auscultates normal and abnormal heart sounds: • $S_1 S_2$ • abnormal heart sounds		Audio tapes	Evaluator confirms identification of heart sounds. Orientee verbalizes possible etiology of abnormal sounds.		
4. Obtains accurate blood pressure readings (systolic and diastolic) utilizing: • manual • automatic		Equipment – manufacturer's instructions	Evaluator confirms accuracy.		
PULMONARY SYSTEM					
Performs a pulmonary assessment and integrates data to determine when a patient is at risk.					
1. Identifies normal breath sounds in anterior, posterior, and lateral lung fields, including vesicular and bronco vesicular breath sounds.		Audio tape	Evaluator confirms auscultatory findings and observes techniques.		

♦ For individuals with prior clinic experience, orientation time frames may be adjusted; however, the minimum competencies must be demonstrated prior to completing orientation. Therefore, the individual may self-assess certain skills that are agreed upon with the clinic nurse, preceptor, charge nurse, or department head.

   ♦ To **self-assess**, write either '**C**' = "competent" or '**ND**' = "needs development" in the "Self-Assess" Column.

♦ In the **'Method to Measure Competency' column**, if the number of times to perform a performance criteria is not stated, it is implied that it will be demonstrated <u>one</u> time.

♦ In the **'Met/Not Met' column** write either **'M'** = "Met" or **'NM'** = "Not Met" and the orienteer's initials. Write specific needs that remain and any other helpful information in the 'comments' column.

DIRECTORATE, PRIMARY CARE

ORIENTATION COMPETENCY STATEMENTS AND PERFORMANCE CRITERIA: Patient Assessment, Education, and Care

COMPETENCY STATEMENT/ PERFORMANCE CRITERIA	SELF-ASSESS	ADDITIONAL LEARNING OPTIONS	METHOD TO MEASURE	M = Met NM = Not Met	COMMENTS
2. Recognizes adventitious breath sounds, including rales (crackles), rhonchi, wheezes, diminished, absent, and unequal.		Audio tape	Evaluator confirms findings on at least 3 patients.		
3. Recognizes abnormal respiratory findings, including: • shallow, irregular breathing • hyperventilation • asymmetrical chest motion • dyspnea/apnea • presence of cyanosis • patient's subjective symptoms (SOB) • use of accessory muscles and abdominal breathing			Evaluator confirms findings and identifies potential causes, treatments, and patient response.		
Provides nursing care for the patient who is unable to maintain a patent airway.					
1. Opens airway. 2. Inserts oral/nasal airway adjunct. 3. Maintains and evaluates effectiveness of airway adjunct.			Evaluator confirms interventions are performed appropriately.		
Provides nursing care for the patient on oxygen therapy.					
1. Identifies rationale for O_2 therapy. 2. Identifies advantages and indications for the following O_2 devices: • Nasal Canula • Face mask • Non re-breather mask 3. Identifies patient conditions/history affecting O2 administration (i.e., COPD). 4. Evaluates effectiveness of O_2 therapy. 5. Obtains accurate pulse oximeter measurements.		Receives in-service on O2 device from evaluator or RT. Observes RN or RT applying oxygen devices and troubleshooting.	Evaluator confirms ability to apply and operate oxygen therapy. Orientee identifies resources to help troubleshoot oxygen devices.		
NEUROLOGICAL SYSTEM					
Performs a neurologic assessment and integrates data to determine when a patient is at risk.					
1. Completes neuro assessment: • level of consciousness/orientation • motor response • strength • reflexes (gag, cough, swallowing)			Evaluator confirms assessment findings. Orientee documents appropriately.		
2. Identifies normal/abnormal neurologic findings, including: • symptoms: headache, LOC changes, weakness, dizziness/visual disturbances, dysphasia,			Evaluator confirms neuro findings. Orientee		

♦ For individuals with prior clinic experience, orientation time frames may be adjusted; however, the minimum competencies must be demonstrated prior to completing orientation. Therefore, the individual may self-assess certain skills that are agreed upon with the clinic nurse, preceptor, charge nurse, or department head.

    ♦ To **self-assess**, write either '**C**' = "competent" or '**ND**' = "needs development" in the "Self-Assess" Column.

♦ In the '**Method to Measure Competency**' column, if the number of times to perform a performance criteria is not stated, it is implied that it will be demonstrated <u>one</u> time.

♦ In the '**Met/Not Met**' column write either '**M**' = "Met" or '**NM**' = "Not Met" and the orienteer's initials. Write specific needs that remain and any other helpful information in the 'comments' column.

DIRECTORATE, PRIMARY CARE

ORIENTATION COMPETENCY STATEMENTS AND PERFORMANCE CRITERIA: **Patient Assessment, Education, and Care**

COMPETENCY STATEMENT/ PERFORMANCE CRITERIA	SELF-ASSESS	ADDITIONAL LEARNING OPTIONS	METHOD TO MEASURE	M = Met NM = Not Met	COMMENTS
ataxia • seizure activity			verbalizes etiology of abnormal findings.		
Provides nursing care for a patient with a neurological deficit.					
1. Completes neurovascular assessment, including: • pupil size • sensation/movement • speech pattern • posturing 2. Aligns patient in proper body positioning. 3. Applies eye protection when indicated. 5. Maintains patient safety, including: • airway protection • seizure precautions • aspiration precautions • fall prevention			Evaluator confirms ability to institute safety measures and prevent complications.		
GASTROINTESTINAL SYSTEM					
Performs a gastrointestinal assessment and integrates data to determine when a patient is at risk.					
1. Identifies normal and abnormal findings: • subjective symptoms: N/V, diarrhea, constipation, pain, dysphasia • inspects abdomen for: distention, symmetry, lesions • auscultates for bowel sounds • palpates abdomen for: rigidity, tenderness, pain • assesses characteristics of BM including amount, color, consistency, presence of blood • assesses characteristics of GI drainage including amount, color, presence of blood • assesses mastication and swallowing ability		Swallowing SLM	Evaluator confirms abdominal assessment. Orientee verbalizes possible etiology for abnormal findings. Orientee completes Swallowing SLM.		
3. Assesses nutritional status: • Recognizes significant unplanned weight loss of more than 5 lbs in the last two months • Inspects skin integrity/skin turgor			Orientee uses resources to identify normal and abnormal findings.		
RENAL SYSTEM					
Performs a renal assessment and integrates data to determine when a patient is at risk.					
1. Identifies normal and abnormal findings, including: • subjective findings: dysuria, urinary frequency, distention • characteristics of urine: volume, color, clarity, presence of blood/sediment, odor			Evaluator confirms assessment findings. Orientee verbalizes possible etiology for		

♦ For individuals with prior clinic experience, orientation time frames may be adjusted; however, the minimum competencies must be demonstrated prior to completing orientation. Therefore, the individual may self-assess certain skills that are agreed upon with the clinic nurse, preceptor, charge nurse, or department head.

    ♦ To **self-assess**, write either '**C**' = "competent" or '**ND**' = "needs development" in the "Self-Assess" Column.

♦ In the '**Method to Measure Competency' column**, if the number of times to perform a performance criteria is not stated, it is implied that it will be demonstrated <u>one</u> time.

♦ In the '**Met/Not Met' column** write either '**M**' = "Met" or '**NM**' = "Not Met" and the orienteer's initials. Write specific needs that remain and any other helpful information in the 'comments' column.

DIRECTORATE, PRIMARY CARE

ORIENTATION COMPETENCY STATEMENTS AND PERFORMANCE CRITERIA: **Patient Assessment, Education, and Care**

COMPETENCY STATEMENT/ PERFORMANCE CRITERIA	SELF-ASSESS	ADDITIONAL LEARNING OPTIONS	METHOD TO MEASURE	M = Met NM = Not Met	COMMENTS
			abnormal findings.		
INTEGUMENTARY SYSTEM					
Performs a skin assessment and integrates data to determine when a patient is at risk.					
1. Performs skin assessment: • Assesses subjective symptoms (itching). • Identifies lesions (rashes), ecchymosis. • Identifies wounds (color, drainage, size). • Identifies and determines stage of pressure ulcers.					
Performs wound/incision care.					
1. Performs wound/incision care per standards, including: • Uses sterile technique. • Uses appropriate antibacterial agents. • Applies appropriate dressing type. 2. Documents wound condition with dressing changes.			Observation.		
PSYCHOSOCIAL ISSUES					
Performs a psychosocial assessment and integrates data to determine when a patient is at risk.					
1. Determines patient's response to the environment, including: • level of anxiety • method of communication • sleep pattern • sensory impaired (hearing, vision, etc.) 2. Identifies patient's psychosocial support system. 3. Assesses patient's coping mechanisms, including previous coping style, culture, and religion. 4. Assesses presence of actual or potential abuse: • identifies physical, psychological or social signs of abuse • accesses appropriate resources • assists with completion of report as needed			Evaluator confirms assessment. Orientee identifies and addresses psychosocial needs in plan of care.		
Controls patient environment according to patient needs.					
1. Assesses fall risk and implements fall precautions as indicated.			Orientee implements		

♦ For individuals with prior clinic experience, orientation time frames may be adjusted; however, the minimum competencies must be demonstrated prior to completing orientation. Therefore, the individual may self-assess certain skills that are agreed upon with the clinic nurse, preceptor, charge nurse, or department head.

   ♦ To **self-assess**, write either 'C' = "competent" or '**ND**' = "needs development" in the "Self-Assess" Column.

♦ In the '**Method to Measure Competency**' column, if the number of times to perform a performance criteria is not stated, it is implied that it will be demonstrated <u>one</u> time.

♦ In the '**Met/Not Met' column** write either '**M**' = "Met" or '**NM**' = "Not Met" and the orienteer's initials. Write specific needs that remain and any other helpful information in the 'comments' column.

DIRECTORATE, PRIMARY CARE

ORIENTATION COMPETENCY STATEMENTS AND PERFORMANCE CRITERIA: **Patient Assessment, Education, and Care**

COMPETENCY STATEMENT/ PERFORMANCE CRITERIA	SELF-ASSESS	ADDITIONAL LEARNING OPTIONS	METHOD TO MEASURE	M = Met NM = Not Met	COMMENTS

• Use of side rails on gurneys
• Providing assistance as needed
  • Utilizing appropriate ambulatory aids, wheelchairs, and approved step stools.
• Identifying potential fall hazards and eliminating (or minimizing and marking) the hazard.
  • Keeping floor and hallways unobstructed and dry.
  • Use of "wet floor" signs.
			interventions directed at controlling patient environment if necessary.
			
			Evaluator confirms patient needs are addressed.		

PAIN MANAGEMENT					
Performs a pain assessment.					
1. Determines patient's acute/chronic pain experience in relation to: • severity (scale 1-10) • location • quality (e.g., burning, sharp, dull) • duration • radiation to other areas • acceptable pain levels • predisposing factors (e.g., activity, coughing and deep breathing, interventions)		AHCPR Guidelines for Acute Pain Management	Evaluator confirms assessment.		
Performs interventions to alleviate/reduce patient's pain.					
1. Explains to patient benefits of effective pain management. 2. Administers pharmacologic therapy appropriately: • Administers analgesics via IM, PO (only Provider or Nurse may administer via IVP or IV infusion). • States benefits and hazards of adjuvant (e.g., benzodiazepines). 3. Provides non-pharmacologic interventions: • Assists patient in splinting • Provides diversionary activities • Relaxation techniques • Pet therapy • Therapeutic touch 4. Evaluates response to treatment.			Evaluator observation.		
PATIENT & FAMILY/SIGNIFICANT OTHER EDUCATION					
Performs a basic educational needs assessment and identifies when a patient and/or family/significant other is at risk.					
1. Assesses learner, including: • abilities (age, past exp., level of knowledge) • readiness to learn • desire and motivation to learn • preferences		Patient/family education standards	Orientee assesses and identifies learning needs of patient/		

♦ For individuals with prior clinic experience, orientation time frames may be adjusted; however, the minimum competencies must be demonstrated prior to completing orientation. Therefore, the individual may self-assess certain skills that are agreed upon with the clinic nurse, preceptor, charge nurse, or department head.

  ♦ To **self-assess**, write either 'C' = "competent" or 'ND' = "needs development" in the "Self-Assess" Column.

♦ In the **'Method to Measure Competency' column**, if the number of times to perform a performance criteria is not stated, it is implied that it will be demonstrated <u>one</u> time.

♦ In the **'Met/Not Met' column** write either **'M'** = "Met" or **'NM'** = "Not Met" and the orienteer's initials. Write specific needs that remain and any other helpful information in the 'comments' column.

DIRECTORATE, PRIMARY CARE

ORIENTATION COMPETENCY STATEMENTS AND PERFORMANCE CRITERIA: Patient Assessment, Education, and Care

COMPETENCY STATEMENT/ PERFORMANCE CRITERIA	SELF-ASSESS	ADDITIONAL LEARNING OPTIONS	METHOD TO MEASURE	M = Met NM = Not Met	COMMENTS
• cultural and religious practices • emotional barriers • physical and cognitive limitations • language barriers • financial implications of care choices • environment 2. Determines presence of knowledge deficit in relation to: • disease process • procedure(s) • medications • medical devices/equipment • diet/nutrition • patient/family responsibilities 3. Verbalizes concepts of adult learning theory.			family/significant other. Evaluator confirms learning needs of patient.		
Provides patient and family/significant other education based on identified needs.					
1. Identifies and prioritizes learning needs based on assessment. 2. Provides individualized instruction, including (as appropriate): • safe and effective use of medications and medical equipment • diet and nutrition (potential drug-food interactions, modified diets) • rights and responsibilities of patient/family (provision of information, compliance with instructions, refusal of treatment, rules and regulations, respect and consideration) • rehabilitation techniques (to assist in adapting and functioning independently in their environment) • personal hygiene and grooming (bathing, brushing teeth, caring for hair/nails, using toilet) • educational resources available in community • follow-up care (when and how to obtain further treatment if needed) 3. Utilizes appropriate educational methods and resources, including: • appropriate members of health care team • education materials (e.g., pamphlets, video, audio) that accommodate patient's unique needs • referral to appropriate programs 4. Evaluates effectiveness of teaching and modifies plan accordingly: • eliciting feedback, questioning • observation, return demonstration		Patient education materials	Evaluator observes patient and family/ significant other education is provided 3 times.		
PROCEDURES					
Demonstrates proficiency in venipuncture. Blood is drawn with minimal discomfort to client. Blood is placed in appropriate tubes and sent to lab.					
1. Demonstrates proper technique in starting peripheral intravenous therapy: • Verifies type of lab test ordered, time for which test is ordered, adequacy of client preparation (fasting state, medication withheld or given).			Evaluator verifies 3 successful		

♦ For individuals with prior clinic experience, orientation time frames may be adjusted; however, the minimum competencies must be demonstrated prior to completing orientation. Therefore, the individual may self-assess certain skills that are agreed upon with the clinic nurse, preceptor, charge nurse, or department head.

♦ To **self-assess**, write either '**C**' = "competent" or '**ND**' = "needs development" in the "Self-Assess" Column.

♦ In the '**Method to Measure Competency**' column, if the number of times to perform a performance criteria is not stated, it is implied that it will be demonstrated <u>one</u> time.

♦ In the '**Met/Not Met** column write either '**M**' = "Met" or '**NM**' = "Not Met" and the orienteer's initials. Write specific needs that remain and any other helpful information in the 'comments' column.

DIRECTORATE, PRIMARY CARE

ORIENTATION COMPETENCY STATEMENTS AND PERFORMANCE CRITERIA: Patient Assessment, Education, and Care

COMPETENCY STATEMENT/ PERFORMANCE CRITERIA	SELF-ASSESS	ADDITIONAL LEARNING OPTIONS	METHOD TO MEASURE	M = Met NM = Not Met	COMMENTS
• Collects and assembles necessary equipment for venipuncture: • vacutainer, sterile needles of appropriate gauge, tourniquet, appropriately colored test tubes • Identifies possible insertion sites. • Preps insertion site. • Performs successful venipunctures safely utilizing age appropriate technique (see Lippincott's: *Nurses' Guide to Clinical Procedures, 4th Ed.*)			venipunctures. Orientee verbalizes: • steps to take if unsuccessful at venipuncture. • possible causes, prevention, and treatment for complications. Orientee demonstrates: • Standard of Care • ability to correctly and safely operate equipment		
Provides nursing care for patients receiving IV therapy.					

1. Identifies rationale for IV therapy.
2. Demonstrates proper technique in starting peripheral intravenous therapy:
  • Collects and assembles necessary equipment for IV insertion/infusion.
  • Verifies IV solution as ordered before administering.
  • Identifies possible insertion sites.
  • Preps insertion site.
  • Performs successful venipunctures safely.
  • Utilizes needleless IV components.
3. Manages peripheral IV catheters/lines (applicable areas), including:
  • Maintains catheter/line patency per standards.
  • Accesses line properly for blood draws, medication administration, and IV infusion.
  • Prevents infection (uses aseptic technique, palpates and inspects insertion site, changes IV tubing and dressing, changes IV solution, changes peripheral IV site, discontinues 16 gauge IV or larger and field IVs within 24° of insertion).
  • Converts venous access device (e.g., IV infusion) to intermittent infusion device (e.g., saline lock).
  • Removes IVs and maintains hemostasis.
		IV P&Ps
		
		Attend IV classes
			Evaluator verifies ability to successfully start 3 PIVs.
			Orientee verbalizes:
			• steps to take if unable to start PIV
			• possible causes, prevention, and treatment for complications
			Orientee demonstrates:
			• Standard of Care in caring for peripheral/ central lines		

♦ For individuals with prior clinic experience, orientation time frames may be adjusted; however, the minimum competencies must be demonstrated prior to completing orientation. Therefore, the individual may self-assess certain skills that are agreed upon with the clinic nurse, preceptor, charge nurse, or department head.

    ♦ To **self-assess**, write either 'C' = "competent" or 'ND' = "needs development" in the "Self-Assess" Column.

    ♦ In the **'Method to Measure Competency' column**, if the number of times to perform a performance criteria is not stated, it is implied that it will be demonstrated <u>one</u> time.

♦ In the **'Met/Not Met' column** write either **'M'** = "Met" or **'NM'** = "Not Met" and the orienteer's initials. Write specific needs that remain and any other helpful information in the 'comments' column.

DIRECTORATE, PRIMARY CARE

ORIENTATION COMPETENCY STATEMENTS AND PERFORMANCE CRITERIA: **Patient Assessment, Education, and Care**

COMPETENCY STATEMENT/ PERFORMANCE CRITERIA	SELF-ASSESS	ADDITIONAL LEARNING OPTIONS	METHOD TO MEASURE	M = Met NM = Not Met	COMMENTS
4. Sets up and maintains IV infusion pump. 5. States potential complications: • infiltration • phlebitis • infection • extravasation			• ability to correctly and safely operate equipment		
Demonstrates proficiency in administering medications.					
1. Ensures written medication order obtained may not receive verbal orders. 2. States the following for each medication listed below: • indications/contraindications • action • dosage (including calculation when appropriate) • side effects • drug compatibility • related nursing care 3. Accurately prepares and administers medications, including: • right patient, drug, dose, route, time 4. Adjusts medications according to specified parameters or as indicated. 5. Evaluates patient's response to medication. 6. Documents medication information appropriately. • Medication administration record, nurses' notes, narcotic sheet, pain flowsheet • Count of controlled drugs at change of shift **Medications:** • Albuterol • Prednisolone • Rocephin • Tylenol • Morphine • Toradol • Phenergan • RhoGAM • Depo-Provera • Glucose (D50, glucagon) • Reversal agents (Narcan, Romazicon)		Consults pharmacist as needed PDR, drug reference P&P – medication administration IV Push Guidelines (corpsman are not permitted to provide anything via IV Push)	Evaluator confirms all medications administered within prescribed time frame. Orientee verbalizes all information to evaluator prior to administering drugs. Evaluator confirms documentation.		

♦ For individuals with prior clinic experience, orientation time frames may be adjusted; however, the minimum competencies must be demonstrated prior to completing orientation. Therefore, the individual may self-assess certain skills that are agreed upon with the clinic nurse, preceptor, charge nurse, or department head.
   ♦ To **self-assess**, write either '**C**' = "competent" or '**ND**' = "needs development" in the "Self-Assess" Column.
♦ In the '**Method to Measure Competency**' column, if the number of times to perform a performance criteria is not stated, it is implied that it will be demonstrated <u>one</u> time.
♦ In the '**Met/Not Met**' column write either '**M**' = "Met" or '**NM**' = "Not Met" and the orienteer's initials. Write specific needs that remain and any other helpful information in the 'comments' column.

DIRECTORATE, PRIMARY CARE

ORIENTATION COMPETENCY STATEMENTS AND PERFORMANCE CRITERIA: Patient Assessment, Education, and Care

COMPETENCY STATEMENT/ PERFORMANCE CRITERIA	SELF-ASSESS	ADDITIONAL LEARNING OPTIONS	METHOD TO MEASURE	M = Met NM = Not Met	COMMENTS
Transfers patient.					
1. SBAR (Situation-Background-Assessment-Recommendation) technique provides a framework for communication between members of the health care team about a patient's condition framing any conversation, especially critical ones, requiring a clinician's immediate attention and action. It allows for an easy and focused way to set expectations for what will be communicated and how between members of the team, which is essential for developing teamwork and fostering a culture of patient safety. 2. Prepares patient for transport. 3. Calls report and informs receiving facility of equipment/special needs. 4. Gathers and transfers paperwork/belongings for transfers (medical record and necessary equipment, patient belongings). 5. Documents according to standards (patient assessment, interventions, treatment). 6. Provides appropriate personnel, equipment, and monitoring during transfer.			Evaluator observation		
Performs documentation according to Standards of Care.					
1. Documents assessment findings, interventions and response to treatment, communication with MD, reason for and effect of PRN medications. 2. Documents patient education.			Evaluator confirms documentation per Standards of Care.		

♦ For individuals with prior clinic experience, orientation time frames may be adjusted; however, the minimum competencies must be demonstrated prior to completing orientation. Therefore, the individual may self-assess certain skills that are agreed upon with the clinic nurse, preceptor, charge nurse, or department head.
   ♦ To **self-assess**, write either 'C' = "competent" or 'ND' = "needs development" in the "Self-Assess" Column.
♦ In the **'Method to Measure Competency' column**, if the number of times to perform a performance criteria is not stated, it is implied that it will be demonstrated <u>one</u> time.
♦ In the **'Met/Not Met' column** write either **'M'** = "Met" or **'NM'** = "Not Met" and the orienteer's initials. Write specific needs that remain and any other helpful information in the 'comments' column.

DIRECTORATE, PRIMARY CARE

ORIENTATION COMPETENCY STATEMENTS AND PERFORMANCE CRITERIA: **Foundational Knowledge**

COMPETENCY STATEMENT/ PERFORMANCE CRITERIA	SELF-ASSESS	ADDITIONAL LEARNING OPTIONS	METHOD TO MEASURE	M = Met NM = Not Met	COMMENTS
Demonstrates knowledge of clinic's SCOPE OF SERVICE.					

1. Demonstrates knowledge of and discusses the scope of services available at the clinic (cross out what is not available):
 ▪ Primary care   • Acute care
 ▪ Physical exams   • Preventive medicine
 ▪ Vasectomy   • Colposcopy
 ▪ Audiograms   • Pharmacy
 ▪ Minor procedures:
    ▪ toenail removal ▪ wart treatment
    ▪ sutures ▪ splints
 ▪ Basic radiological and laboratory exams
		Directorate Primary Care SOP	Orienteer verbalization.		

Demonstrates BEHAVIORS OF A PROFESSIONAL.					
1. Maintains patient's rights, dignity, well-being, and confidentiality. 2. Communicates, effectively, information with patient/family/significant other, co-workers, physicians, support services. 3. Recognizes responsibility and accountability for providing quality care: • actual/potential problem identification • problem resolution • channels for communication 4. Summarizes organization's mission, values, and philosophy (MVP). 5. Describes and discusses the roles and responsibilities of position assigned. 6. Discusses patient rights/responsibilities. 7. Describes patient advocacy role. 8. Incorporates spiritual and cultural aspects when caring for specific populations. 9. Demonstrates customer service behaviors to:		Organizations mission, values, and philosophy Patient Rights & Responsibilities Document P&P: Ethical Issues Customer Service Handout	Evaluator observation. Orienteer verbalization.		

◆ For individuals with prior clinic experience, orientation time frames may be adjusted however; the minimum competencies must be demonstrated prior to completing orientation. Therefore, the individual may self-assess certain skills that are agreed upon with the clinic nurse and/or Division Officer.
  ◆ To **self-assess**, write either **'C'** = "competent" or **'ND'** = "needs development" in the "Self-Assess" Column.
◆ In the **'Method to Measure Competency' column**, if the number of times to perform a performance criterion is not stated, it is implied that it will be demonstrated <u>one</u> time.
◆ In the **'Met/Not Met' column** write either **'M'** = "Met" or **'NM'** = "Not Met" and the orienteer's initials. Write specific needs that remain and any other helpful information in the 'comments' column.

DIRECTORATE, PRIMARY CARE

ORIENTATION COMPETENCY STATEMENTS AND PERFORMANCE CRITERIA: Foundational Knowledge

COMPETENCY STATEMENT/ PERFORMANCE CRITERIA	SELF-ASSESS	ADDITIONAL LEARNING OPTIONS	METHOD TO MEASURE	M = Met NM = Not Met	COMMENTS

• patient/family/significant others
• physicians
• interdisciplinary team members
• co-workers
• community
10. Identifies resources for issues related to:
   • ethical concerns
   • patient rights/responsibilities
   • advance directives
   • quality activities					

Demonstrates knowledge of how to provide exceptional CUSTOMER SERVICE.					

1. Demonstrates appropriate courtesies.
    ■ Use of "magic phrases"
      ■ please
      ■ thank you
      ■ you're welcome
      ■ person's rank/title/name
      ■ I'm sorry
    ■ Answer or call promptly
    ■ Identify self clearly
    ■ Listen carefully
    ■ Take accurate notes
    ■ Convey sincere interest and concern
    ■ Agree as often as possible
    ■ Remain calm and courteous
    ■ Avoid interruptions
      ■ Avoid placing the blame
      ■ Avoid making the impression of "passing the buck"
		Attend customer service training	Evaluator observation.
			
			Orienteer verbalization.		

♦ For individuals with prior clinic experience, orientation time frames may be adjusted however; the minimum competencies must be demonstrated prior to completing orientation. Therefore, the individual may self-assess certain skills that are agreed upon with the clinic nurse and/or Division Officer.

  ♦ To **self-assess**, write either **'C'** = "competent" or **'ND'** = "needs development" in the "Self-Assess" Column.

♦ In the **'Method to Measure Competency' column**, if the number of times to perform a performance criterion is not stated, it is implied that it will be demonstrated <u>one</u> time.

♦ In the **'Met/Not Met' column** write either **'M'** = "Met" or **'NM'** = "Not Met" and the orienteer's initials. Write specific needs that remain and any other helpful information in the 'comments' column.

DIRECTORATE, PRIMARY CARE

ORIENTATION COMPETENCY STATEMENTS AND PERFORMANCE CRITERIA: **Foundational Knowledge**

COMPETENCY STATEMENT/ PERFORMANCE CRITERIA	SELF-ASSESS	ADDITIONAL LEARNING OPTIONS	METHOD TO MEASURE	M = Met NM = Not Met	COMMENTS
▪ Avoids personal contact ▪ Follow through					
Demonstrates knowledge of role during EMERGENCY RESPONSES.					
1. Demonstrates knowledge of and procedures to perform during: ▪ Code Blue: Cardiac arrest, unresponsive individual ▪ Code Red: Fire ▪ Code White: Unruly or combative individual ▪ Code Purple: Disaster threat/situation ▪ Code Pink: Abducted infant/child ▪ Code Green: Helicopter			Evaluator observation. Orienteer verbalization.		
Demonstrates appropriate use of COMMUNICATION SYSTEMS.					
1. Demonstrates appropriate use of the clinic's Public Announcement (PA) system. 2. Demonstrates appropriate use of telephone system. 3. Demonstrates appropriate use of the computer systems (Electronic Health Record [HER], OUTLOOK, Internet Explorer, Windows Explorer): <u>Windows Explorer</u> • Sign on/out • "Secure" computer when away from desk <u>EHR</u> • Front desk menu • Review clinical results • Orders menu • Print medical note • Immunizations menu • Schedules and Templates <u>IT</u> • Read e-mail • Perform search of files		Documentation Standards of Care Completes Administrative Procedure, fire safety, safety, infection control, hazardous material, general utility failures, mass casualty, physical security of unit competencies	Orienteer: ▪ Books at least 3 appointments ▪ enters 3 walk-ins ▪ prints modified note ▪ displays results for lab, x-ray, C&S ▪ enters immunizations for 3 records, prints history and physical short and long format ▪ Locates clinic's		

♦ For individuals with prior clinic experience, orientation time frames may be adjusted however; the minimum competencies must be demonstrated prior to completing orientation. Therefore, the individual may self-assess certain skills that are agreed upon with the clinic nurse and/or Division Officer.

   ♦ To **self-assess**, write either **'C'** = "competent" or **'ND'** = "needs development" in the "Self-Assess" Column.

♦ In the **'Method to Measure Competency' column**, if the number of times to perform a performance criterion is not stated, it is implied that it will be demonstrated <u>one</u> time.

♦ In the **'Met/Not Met' column** write either **'M'** = "Met" or **'NM'** = "Not Met" and the orienteer's initials. Write specific needs that remain and any other helpful information in the 'comments' column.

DIRECTORATE, PRIMARY CARE

ORIENTATION COMPETENCY STATEMENTS AND PERFORMANCE CRITERIA: **Foundational Knowledge**

COMPETENCY STATEMENT/ PERFORMANCE CRITERIA	SELF-ASSESS	ADDITIONAL LEARNING OPTIONS	METHOD TO MEASURE	M = Met NM = Not Met	COMMENTS

• Clinic's share drive
• Intranet: safety info, reference sites, phone book, higher authority instructions, departmental Web pages, and other pertinent information
4. Demonstrates how to access and the appropriate use of pager system.
5. Demonstrates appropriate use of fax machine.
6. Demonstrates appropriate use of copier machine.
7. Initiates and completes incident report.
8. Locates reference manuals in clinic's intranet and share drive.
  • Directorate Primary Care (DPC) SOP • Clinic specific SOPs
  • Disaster Preparedness & Response Plan • Safety SOP
  • Infection Control SOP • MSDS
  • Lippincott's Complete Nursing Reference • Micro-Medix
  • Nurses' Guide to Clinical Procedures • Telelibrary
9. Locates and demonstrates appropriate use of emergency systems:
  ▪ Fire call box, extinguishers, exits
  ▪ Code Blue, Code Red, Code Pink, Code Purple, Code White, Code Green
			electronic folders for SOP, Instructions Intranet and resource links
			
			Evaluator observation		

Demonstrates knowledge of SAFETY standards and procedures.					
1. Demonstrates knowledge of situations when Personal Protective Equipment (PPE) is required and demonstrates proper care, donning, and use. 2. Demonstrates proper handling and disposal of sharps and biohazard materials. 3. States when sharp containers are to be replaced and how to properly package and label the full sharp container for transport to USNH. 4. States what should and should not be discarded in a biohazard bag/container. 5. Demonstrates knowledge of Environment of Care standards. ▪ Clinic layout, location of emergency exits, fire extinguishers/alarms, and muster location		Safety Manual	Evaluator observation. Orienteer verbalization.		

♦ For individuals with prior clinic experience, orientation time frames may be adjusted however; the minimum competencies must be demonstrated prior to completing orientation. Therefore, the individual may self-assess certain skills that are agreed upon with the clinic nurse and/or Division Officer.
  ♦ To **self-assess**, write either '**C**' = "competent" or '**ND**' = "needs development" in the "Self-Assess" Column.
♦ In the **'Method to Measure Competency' column**, if the number of times to perform a performance criterion is not stated, it is implied that it will be demonstrated <u>one</u> time.
♦ In the **'Met/Not Met' column** write either '**M**' = "Met" or '**NM**' = "Not Met" and the orienteer's initials. Write specific needs that remain and any other helpful information in the 'comments' column.

DIRECTORATE, PRIMARY CARE

ORIENTATION COMPETENCY STATEMENTS AND PERFORMANCE CRITERIA: **Foundational Knowledge**

COMPETENCY STATEMENT/ PERFORMANCE CRITERIA	SELF-ASSESS	ADDITIONAL LEARNING OPTIONS	METHOD TO MEASURE	M = Met NM = Not Met	COMMENTS
▪ Appropriate response and actions to take during Codes Blue, Red, White, Green, Purple, and Pink ▪ Appropriate storage, handling and disposal of HazMat used ▪ Response and reporting procedures for mishaps and unsafe/unhealthful working conditions ▪ Completed site specific safety training and appropriate medical surveillances					
Demonstrates knowledge of INFECTION CONTROL standards and procedures per the Infection Control Manual.					
1. Demonstrates knowledge of Universal Precautions. 2. Discusses and demonstrates proper handling and removal/disposal of contaminated linen, equipment, and supplies. 3. Demonstrates knowledge of proper cleaning of equipment and work areas. 4. Demonstrates knowledge of isolation precautions and procedures: 　▪ Airborne precautions 　　▪ Tuberculosis　　▪ Measles▪ Varicella 　▪ Droplet precautions 　　▪ Certain types of meningitis and pneumonia　　▪ Pertussis 　　▪ Influenza　　▪ German measles 　▪ Contact precautions 　　▪ Herpes　　▪ Impetigo　▪ Diphtheria 　　▪ Clostridium difficile　▪ Scabies　▪ MRSA 5. Response and reporting procedures for blood borne pathogen exposures.		Infection Control Manual http://www.cdc.gov/ncidod/	Evaluator observation. Orienteer verbalization.		
Demonstrates knowledge of the confines of their certifications, licenses, privileges/credentials, and practices within.					
1. Demonstrates knowledge of the certifications/training to obtain and maintain: 　▪ Providers: BLS, ACLS, PALS, NALs, ATLS, RSI			Orienteer verbalization.		

◆ For individuals with prior clinic experience, orientation time frames may be adjusted however; the minimum competencies must be demonstrated prior to completing orientation. Therefore, the individual may self-assess certain skills that are agreed upon with the clinic nurse and/or Division Officer.
　◆ To **self-assess**, write either '**C**' = "competent" or '**ND**' = "needs development" in the "Self-Assess" Column.
◆ In the **'Method to Measure Competency' column**, if the number of times to perform a performance criterion is not stated, it is implied that it will be demonstrated <u>one</u> time.
◆ In the **'Met/Not Met' column** write either **'M'** = "Met" or **'NM'** = "Not Met" and the orienteer's initials. Write specific needs that remain and any other helpful information in the 'comments' column.

DIRECTORATE, PRIMARY CARE

ORIENTATION COMPETENCY STATEMENTS AND PERFORMANCE CRITERIA: Foundational Knowledge

COMPETENCY STATEMENT/ PERFORMANCE CRITERIA	SELF-ASSESS	ADDITIONAL LEARNING OPTIONS	METHOD TO MEASURE	M = Met NM = Not Met	COMMENTS
▪ Nurses: BLS, TNCC, ACLS, PALS, NALs, Medication, IV, Immunizations 2. Verbalizes knowledge of: ▪ Not accept or act upon verbal orders ▪ May not push IV medications ▪ May not administer medications until med certified ▪ May not suture without direct supervision until suture certified ▪ May not administer immunizations unless immunization certified ▪ IV Conscious Sedation may not be performed in the clinic					
2009 National Patient Safety Goals					
1. Demonstrates Universal Protocol. 2. Improve the accuracy of patient identification. 3. Improve the effectiveness of communication among caregivers. 4. Improve the safety of using medications. 5. Reduce the risk of health care associated infections. 6. Accurately and completely reconcile medications across the continuum of care. 7. Reduce the risk of surgical fires. 8. Encourage patients' active involvement in their own care as a patient safety strategy.					

- ◆ For individuals with prior clinic experience, orientation time frames may be adjusted however; the minimum competencies must be demonstrated prior to completing orientation. Therefore, the individual may self-assess certain skills that are agreed upon with the clinic nurse and/or Division Officer.
  - ◆ To **self-assess**, write either '**C**' = "competent" or '**ND**' = "needs development" in the "Self-Assess" Column.
- ◆ In the **'Method to Measure Competency' column**, if the number of times to perform a performance criterion is not stated, it is implied that it will be demonstrated <u>one</u> time.
- ◆ In the **'Met/Not Met' column** write either **'M'** = "Met" or **'NM'** = "Not Met" and the orienteer's initials. Write specific needs that remain and any other helpful information in the 'comments' column.

MeritCare Health System
Initial Orientation Competency Verification Checklist
Ambulatory RN/LPN

Name _____ Title _____ Start Date _____ Service Area _____ Primary Preceptor _____

Directions: This checklist includes the **high-risk/high-frequency** processes/clinical skills and emergency response for this job.

Associate:
- Complete the self-assessment during Nursing Orientation – **Self-Assessment Codes: F** = Frequently **I** = Infrequently **N** = Never
- Review the **MeritCare** policy or other pertinent resource prior to performing. **Frequently used resources:** Potter & Perry – Nursing Fundamentals; Patient Care, Infection Control, and Patient Education Manuals in CareNet.

Preceptors:
- Assist in locating/reviewing policies and other resources prior to performing the skill.
- Place a √ in the box when the new nurse **PRACTICES/PERFORMS** the skill.
- **VALIDATE COMPETENCY** by **Dating/Initialing** when the associate can complete the skill safely, legally, and correctly with minimal coaching.
- Ensure all skills are signed off or have an "N/A." Write "N/A" if not applicable for this area. **Observation is the preferred verification method.** If unable to observe, then either (S) simulate, (C) use a critical thinking scenario, or validate through (CR) chart review.
- Document full signature one time at end of form.

Manager: When checklist is complete, verify completion of orientation by dating and signing and send to Learning Services.

Patient Populations Served (check all that apply):
Neonate (<1mo)   Infants (1mo-1yr)   Child (age 1-12)   Adolescent (13-17)   Adult (18-64)   Geriatric (65 +)

At completion of Orientation: Send copy to Learning Services #376 for employee record as soon as orientation is complete or within 90 days of hire. Retain a copy in Service Area file also.

Clinical Competencies/Skills	Self-Assessment: I have performed this skill.			Reviewed in Nursing Orientation	Competence Verification (Preceptor Initials) by Week: Date/Preceptor Initials = Validating Competency							
	F	I	N		1	2	3	4	5	6	7	8
SERVICE EXCELLENCE												
Service Excellence Commitments												
Answering phones/phone etiquette												
"Is there anything else I can do for you? I have the time."												
ASSESSMENT OF PATIENT												
Pt. encounter with provider												
New pt./annual/ pre-op visits												
PLANNING CARE/NURSING DIAGNOSIS												
DIAGNOSTIC TESTING												
Audiogram-age appropriate (Welch/Allyn, Pilot)												
Vision Screening (include color testing)												
Perform 12 Lead EKG												
Performs Stress Test												
Performs Peak Flowmeter												
Communication of Critical test results												
Point of Care Competencies (lab)												
PRIORITIZATION/ ORGANIZATION/TRIAGE												
EVALUATING OUTCOMES												
PATIENT EDUCATION												
Utilizes Teach-back method												
Uses pt. ed./Equal Access resources												
Uses Centricity – pt. ed. handouts												
Documentation of pt. education												

Competency Verification (Preceptor Initials) by Week:
√ = Practices/Performs
Date/Preceptor Initials = Validating Competency

Clinical Competencies/Skills	Self-Assessment: I have performed this skill.			Reviewed in Nursing Orientation	Competence Verification (Preceptor Initials) by Week: √ = Practices/Performs Date/Preceptor Initials = Validating Competency							
	F	I	N		1	2	3	4	5	6	7	8
DOCUMENTATION												
Physician Orders/verification												
No Dangerous abbreviations												
Date and Time ALL documentation and orders (all who document in pt. record)												
TORBV and VORBV – MD sign off in 48 hrs												
Utilizes electronic medical record												
Enter phone note												
Enter order												
Enter treatment letter												
Enter lab order												
Send flags												
Convert a flag to a phone note												
Work from a co-worker's desktop												
ABN Form												
PATIENT SAFETY												
Patient Identifiers-what/when required												
Labeling lab specimens												
Time-out for procedures												
Critical Test Results												
Look alike/Sound alike meds and high risk meds – aware of												
Site Marking by physician/provider												
Restraints												
Monitors patient in restraints/documents												
Patient Handoffs												
Uses SBAR												
Family Communication (Password)												
Medication Management												
Medication Administration – 6 rights												
Completes list of current meds												
Med Reconciliation												
Provides pt. with updated med list												
Labels medications/solutions on/off sterile field												
Secure/appropriate storage of meds												
Monitor refrigerator/freezer temp												
Knowledgeable about med before administering												
Monitors effects of medications												
Routes: IVPB, IV Push, Opthalmic, Topical, Oral												
Intramuscular												
Ventrogluteal site IM												
Subcutaneous												
Immunizations												
Allergy Serum												
Mantoux												
Anticoagulation therapy – policy												
Irrigation – Eye/Ear												
IV Infusion Pump												

Clinical Competencies/Skills	Self-Assessment: I have performed this skill.			Reviewed in Nursing Orientation	Competence Verification (Preceptor Initials) by Week: √ = Practices/Performs Date/Preceptor Initials = Validating Competency							
	F	I	N		1	2	3	4	5	6	7	8
Infection Control-Reducing Health Care Associated Infections												
Hand Hygiene												
Triages pts. with infectious diseases												
Contact Precautions: MRSA, VRE				▓								
Tests Cidex OPA												
Cleans/Disinfects equipment												
Sterile procedures												
Set-up sterile tray/instruments												
Preps pt./demonstrates sterile scrub												
Safe Patient Handling & Mobility (SPHM)												
Gait belts												
Ambulation – crutches, walker				▓								
Application/Assessment of splints/slings												
INTEGUMENTARY												
Staple/suture removal												
Sterile dressing changes												
EMERGENCIES												
Early recognition of cues/status change				▓								
BLS status current				▓								
Crash Cart location/Emergency bag				▓								
Assembles/applies pocket mask/ambu												
Locate/Check AED												
Initiate emergency response/CPR												
Code Team Roles/Site-specific protocols												
NEUROLOGICAL												
Recognizes signs of stroke												
GASTROINTESTINAL/GENITOURINARY												
Bladder Scanner – interprets												
Collects specimens												
Insertion/removal of urinary catheter												
CARDIOVASCULAR/RESPIRATORY												
B/P												
Venipuncture				▓								
Central Venous Access												
Sterile dressing change with medication impregnated dressing				▓								
Flushes				▓								
Draws blood												
Discontinues (RN only)												
Accesses Port (RN only)												
PAIN MANAGEMENT												
Assessment/Reassessment				▓								
Referral as appropriate				▓								
Additional High Risk/Frequency Competency/Skills for Patient Population												

251

Preceptor Comments:

I verify this associate has met the minimum competencies for their position, and high-risk and high-frequency skills have been verified. The initial assessment of competency is complete.

Initials & Verification Signatures:

_____   _____   _____
                                        Date   Manager/Reviewer

Original Implementation date: 12/04 Content Revision: 10/05, 9/06, 10/08

	RN	LPN
Assessment	CONDUCTS AND DOCUMENTS nursing assessments, validating, refining, and modifying data.	CONTRIBUTES TO the assessment of health status of patients by collecting basic objective and subjective data, assisting in validating, refining, and modifying the data.
Diagnosis	ANALYZES the assessment data to establish or modify nursing diagnosis.	CONTRIBUTES TO establishing nursing diagnoses that identify the needs of the patient.
Planning	In collaboration with the patient, DEVELOPS a plan of care based on nursing assessment and diagnosis that prescribes interventions to attain expected outcomes. Identifies community resources needed for continued care and makes referrals.	PARTICIPATES IN the development of the plan of care for individuals.
Implementation	IMPLEMENTS the plan of care and the nursing interventions, determining the responsibilities that can properly and safely be assigned or delegated.	PARTICIPATES IN implementing nursing plan of care and nursing interventions by caring for patients who are stable or predictable; delegating or assigning components of nursing care to other members of the nursing care team.
Evaluation	EVALUATES the responses to nursing interventions, modifying nursing diagnoses, revising strategies of care, and prescribing changes in nursing interventions.	CONTRIBUTES TO the evaluation of the responses of individuals to nursing interventions, assisting in modifying the plan of care based upon the evaluation.
Documentation	Thoroughly documents patient information.	Thoroughly documents patient information.
Patient Education	ASSESSES patient needs and designs; implements and evaluates a teaching plan.	ASSISTS WITH the assessment of patient needs. Provides patient teaching according to the developed plan.

COMMUNITY MEMORIAL MEDICAL COMMONS
PRIMARY CARE INITIATIVE
Internal Medicine Registered Nurse (RN) Skills/Competency Checklist

EMPLOYEE: _____ DATE OF HIRE/TRANSFER: _____ SUPERVISOR: _____

The Skills/Competency Checklist is a tool used to document demonstrated ability in all patient care skills and general duties. It is a guide to becoming an effective, efficient, and competent employee. Skills may be demonstrated to and signed off by another RN, Physician, or Supervisor as appropriate. It is your responsibility to ensure that all skills assessments are completed and documented. Experiences are available in many areas of the department. The Skills Checklist should be completed within the first three months of employment or transfer and submitted to the clinic supervisor upon completion. The original will be filed in your Personnel Record.

STANDARD COMPETENCY	Date Reviewed/ Observer Initials	Date Demonstrated/ Observer Initials	Completed Date and Observer Signature
1. Demonstrates appropriate and efficient use of department specific equipment/software necessary to perform role (multi-feature telephones, call distribution, keyboard skills, Windows and call processing software, EPIC, modem, fax, copier, etc.): 1.1 Demonstrates knowledge and skill to correctly log onto telephone system, initiate and complete transfers, paging, etc. 1.2 Demonstrates knowledge and skill to navigate in Windows. 1.3 Demonstrates knowledge and skill to navigate in EPIC. 1.4 Demonstrates proficient use of Windows Outlook and EPIC InBasket. 1.5 Demonstrates proficiency in releasing clinic charges in EPIC.			
2. Demonstrates positive telephone interaction skills as evidenced by: 2.1 Courteousness (identifies self, refers to caller by name, pleasant tone of voice, allows caller to express issue, etc.). 2.2 Speaks directly to individual with symptoms whenever possible.			

W129 N7055 Northfield Dr., Building A, Suite 100
Menomonee Falls, Wisconsin 53051

2.3 Asks open-ended questions to identify actual or potential health problems.			
2.4 Restates problem to verify congruency with patient/caller's perception.			
2.5 Uses lay terminology with providing explanations and instructions.			
2.6 Focuses conversations for goal-directed, time-limited communication.			
2.7 Offers caller opportunity to express any concerns/ problems before ending call.			
2.8 Maintains professional composure in high stress, emotional situations.			
2.9 Maintains confidentiality of all interactions.			
2.10 Follows process/call management guides specific to the client population.			
2.11 Documents all telephone contact with patients in EPIC as a telephone encounter.			
3. Complies with call management standard benchmarks as evidenced by our Press Ganey scores: 3.1 Our helpfulness on the telephone—Our Goal is 85%. 3.2 Our promptness in returning calls—Our Goal is 65%. 3.3 Ease of getting clinic on phone—Our Goal is 70%. 3.4 Availability of care provider to talk on phone—Our Goal is 75%.			
4. Demonstrates appropriate management and paper documentation of calls if computer system is down.			
5. Complies with department and organizational policies and procedures related to: 5.1 Managing emergency medical system or crisis intervention referrals. 5.2 Confidentiality of all patient encounters (HIPAA). 5.3 Safety practices required by nature to work (infection control, risk			

W129 N7055 Northfield Dr., Building A, Suite 100
Menomonee Falls, Wisconsin 53051

management, etc.). 5.4 Reporting of incidents (patient or employee). 5.5 Risk management procedures (med. admin., equipment malfunction reporting, removal of specs from exam room prior to bringing in another patient). 5.6 Mandated reporting policies.			
6. Demonstrates concern for cost-effective operations by working productively to reduce inefficiencies: 6.1 Meets attendance standards. 6.2 Consistently reports to work on time. 6.3 Uses time productively by coordinating tasks, avoiding excessive socialization, completing timely work, and using slow time to department advantage. 6.4 Agrees to work flexible schedule as needed which is based on provider needs. 6.5 Assists team members as needed without prompting. 6.6 Requests coaching and assistance from preceptors/other experienced staff when needed. 6.7 Demonstrates multitasking of duties for the efficient running of providers' clinic.			
7. Able to express clearly the nature and scope of the CMMC/PCI clinic including, but not limited to: 7.1 Define mission of service. 7.2 Describe client populations served by clinic.			
8. Daily operations within POD and Clinic: 8.1 Rooming of patients according to established standards 8.2 Clinic set-up – Start of day process. 8.3 Verbalizes MA/LPN/RN role in clinic. 8.4 Verbalizes registration, arrival and check-out process. 8.5 Specimen handling and labeling. 8.6 Supplies – Ordering and stocking process. 8.7 Disposition and prioritization of calls.			

W129 N7055 Northfield Dr., Building A, Suite 100
Menomonee Falls, Wisconsin 53051

8.8   Paging staff.
8.9   Personal protective equipment.
8.10 Performs POCT according to established guidelines:
    8.101 12 lead Electrocardiogram
    8.102 Peak flow
    8.103 Spirometry
    8.104 Glucometer
    8.105 Rapid Influenza
    8.106 Rapid Strep A
    8.107 Monospot
    8.108 Urinalysis
    8.109 Urine Pregnancy
    8.110 Rapid RSV testing
    8.111 Snellen Test			

9.   Performs and/or assists with procedures according to guidelines and specific to the clinic, including appropriate documentation of the following:
Upon MD order, performs independently:
    9.1   Ear lavage
    9.2   Suture removal
    9.3   Obtaining nasopharyngeal and throat swabs
    9.4   Interdermal and subcutaneous injections
    9.5   Administration of vaccines
    9.6   Nebulizers
Assistance with the following:
    9.7   Incision and drainage
    9.8   Laceration repair
    9.9   Mole removal
    9.10 Pap smears
    9.11 Punch biopsy
    9.12 Sterile technique
    9.13 Steroid injection			

9.14 Toe nail removal			
9.15 Wart removal			
9.16 Assist with local anesthetic administration			
REGISTERED NURSE CORE COMPETENCY			

10.   Using nursing knowledge and skill, performs telephone triage by managing clinical calls using the nursing process:
   10.1 Assesses life-threatening or crisis situations at onset of a call and manages the referral to EMS.
   10.2 Records the caller's presenting problem; include specific quote of caller perception of the problem, its onset, severity, duration, and any other current symptoms.
   10.3 Assesses and documents relevant clinical profile of the caller for current situation, including diagnosed health problems, recent infections/reactions, health risks.
   10.4 Demonstrates critical thinking by assessing covert as well as overt parameters relevant to the needs of the caller.
   10.5 Establishes priorities (prioritizing incoming calls and disposition of calls). Able to reprioritize as situation requires.
   10.6 Based on assessed information, accurately determines the most appropriate triage guideline for the situation.
   10.7 Uses additional references when needed to meet the needs of the caller.
   10.8 Demonstrates knowledge of clinic and community resources available to meet caller needs.
   10.9 Utilizes clinical assessment of caller variables to maintain appropriateness of disposition (defined urgency) with availability of clinical service (provider office, urgent care, ED, etc.).
   10.10 Provides care advice to caller specific to their needs.
   10.11 Evaluates and documents the caller's intended action.
   10.12 Closes call by allowing caller to express resolution of expressed needs and /or additional needs/concerns.			

10.13 Schedules call back for caller as defined by need and/or policy. 10.14 Complies with nursing scope of practice for the state of Wisconsin. 10.15 Assists with clinic flow and workload management.			

11. Documents caller(patient) encounters in the system that are:
  11.1 Entered concurrently with encounter.
  11.2 Uses appropriate and correctly spelled medical terminology.
  11.3 Reflective of assessed needs, recommended action, Understanding, and intended response of caller for each interaction.
  11.4 Reflects plan of care specific to the actual or potential health needs of the caller.			

12. Documents clinic (patient) interactions, nursing interventions, and release of charges done in the clinic.
  12.1 Any patient teaching done
  12.2 Any patient intervention
  12.3 "Release" any changes associated with specific "Smart Set" Orders.			

13. Medication refill according to established medication refill guidelines.
  13.1 Locates fax sent from pharmacy either on fax machine or in according folder.
  13.2 Determine type of medication and refer to clinic list of "No auto fax medications" to identify how to move forward.
  13.3 Determine right patient.
  13.4 View patient medication list/history in EPIC.
  13.5 Determine need for labs or f/u appointment.
  13.6 Refill medication either for present month, 3 months, or a year based on above investigation and protocol.
  13.7 Pend and then route those medications not to be auto faxed, based on protocol.
  13.8 Authorize medication refills for 3 months, notifying pharmacist			

W129 N7055 Northfield Dr., Building A, Suite 100
Menomonee Falls, Wisconsin 53051

refill stipulation is that patient needs to call clinic and make an appointment (medication/situations based on P&P). 13.9 Call patient to inform refill restriction and necessary lab work/appointment needed in order to justify continuation of refill. 13.10 Schedule an appointment.			
14. Performs clinical skill within scope of practice and according to evidence based practice guidelines, being a role model to the clinic UAP as evidenced by: 14.1 Demonstrates sound infection control processes involving the demonstration of universal/standard precautions. 14.2 Demonstrates accurate vital sign measurements, knowledge of abnormalities and uses critical thinking skills to determine if abnormalities are critical and need immediate reporting. 14.3 Assess pain according to evidence based practice guidelines/standards. 14.4 Demonstrates the safe set-up of clinic equipment such as oxygen tanks. 14.5 Performs IV insertion and medication administration according to established nursing care standards and documents interventions accurately. 14.6 Demonstrates and documents wound assessment and wound care according to established guidelines. 14.7 Demonstrates and documents insertion and removal of foley catheter according to established standards. 14.8 Demonstrates and documents general principles and concepts of pre- and post-op teaching using the combination of the nursing process, knowledge of general and specific operative procedures, and finally, adult learning theory.			

W129 N7055 Northfield Dr., Building A, Suite 100
Menomonee Falls, Wisconsin 53051

Signature: _____	Initials: _____	Date: _____	
Signature: _____	Initials: _____	Date: _____	
Signature: _____	Initials: _____	Date: _____	
Signature: _____	Initials: _____	Date: _____	
Signature: _____	Initials: _____	Date: _____	
Signature: _____	Initials: _____	Date: _____	
Signature: _____	Initials: _____	Date: _____	

W129 N7055 Northfield Dr., Building A, Suite 100
Menomonee Falls, Wisconsin 53051

Our member benefits give you the opportunity to...

- ## Discover and network
  Attend AAACN's Annual Conference:
  Top experts and dynamic sessions on the latest innovations in nursing practice. Networking, continuing education credit, special member rates.

- ## Lead and advocate
  Experience the rewards of volunteering:
  Influence the future of ambulatory care nursing. Serve at the national level; join special interest groups, task forces, and committees; start or participate in Local Networking Groups.

- ## Learn and grow
  Access the industry's best publications: Members receive *ViewPoint*, AAACN's award-winning newsletter, your pipeline to advances in practice, news, and resources. Membership also includes an additional subscription to a leading nursing journal of your choice and our monthly e-newsletter.

Additional benefits:

- Discounts on a vast array of education opportunities, services, learning tools, and specialty publications (visit www.aaacn.org).

- Scholarships, research grants, and awards.

- Member-focused Web site (www.aaacn.org) - forums, chat rooms, electronic mailing lists, career center. Access to experts to answer your practice questions.

- Membership directory - network with members across the country.

- Choice of membership in a Special Interest Group. Visit www.aaacn.org for a complete listing.

"The organization provides a variety of information on the many aspects of ambulatory care. The conferences are wonderful."

— Reneil Milewski, BSN, RN

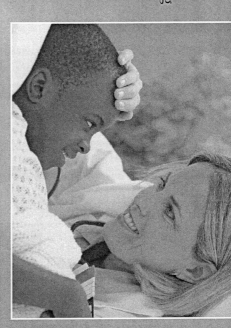

Their practice settings

- Group practices/health centers
- Military and government institutions
- University hospitals
- Community/private hospitals
- Managed care/HMOs/PPOs
- Public sector/community health centers
- Free-standing facilities
- Universities/colleges/educational institutions

Our members

- Nurse managers and supervisors
- Nursing administrators and directors
- Staff nurses
- Educators
- Consultants
- Nurse Practitioners
- Researchers

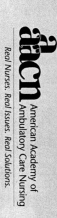

American Academy of Ambulatory Care Nursing

Real Nurses, Real Issues, Real Solutions.

East Holly Avenue/Box 56, Pitman, New Jersey 08071-0056
1-800-AMB-NURS (262-6877) • Fax: 856-589-7463 • www.aaacn.org • E-mail: aaacn@aji.com

ANNUAL CONFERENCE

Hear nationally known speakers who present the latest information on a wide range of ambulatory nursing topics. You are sure to find sessions that will challenge and inspire you. The Annual Conference is held in the spring of each year.

Visit www.aaacn.org/conference for information on upcoming AAACN conferences.

aaacn

American Academy of Ambulatory Care Nursing

Real Nurses. Real Issues. Real Solutions.

1-800-AMB-NURS • Web site: www.aaacn.org • E-mail: aaacn@ajj.com

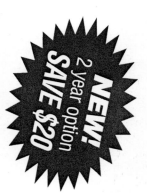

NEW! 2 year option SAVE $20

AAACN Membership Application

M10K

Membership Fee

Dues are not deductible as a charitable organization, but may qualify as a business expense.

Categories of Membership (Please check one)

☐ **Active (RN)** **$130**
Available to any registered nurse.

☐ **LPN/LVN** **$105**

☐ **Active (RN)** **$240**
Pay 2 years – *SAVE $20!*

☐ **Senior** **$70**
Active member for 3 years and reached age 62.

☐ **Affiliate** **$105**
Professional interested in ambulatory care nursing.

☐ **Student** **$70**
Course of study for initial licensure - enclose proof of enrollment.

☐ Check payable in US Funds to AAACN
☐ Charge my ☐ Visa ☐ MasterCard ☐ AmEx

Card # _____

3 or 4 digit security code _____

Expiration Date _____ in the amount of $ _____

Card Holder (print): _____

Credit card billing address: (street number only) _____

Zip Code _____

Signature _____

Name: _____ Credentials: _____

Preferred Mailing Address (check one)

☐ **Home**

Home Address: _____

City: _____ State: _____ Zip: _____

Home Phone: ( ) _____

☐ **Employer:**

Work Address: _____

Employer: _____

City: _____ State: _____ Zip: _____

Business Phone: ( ) _____ Fax #: ( ) _____

Preferred Daytime Phone: ☐ Home ☐ Work

E-mail: _____

AAACN **does not** sell or share member e-mail addresses with any outside parties. It is extremely important for us to have your e-mail address to send your dues renewal notice, monthly E-newsletters, and other timely information.

Fax this form to (856) 589-7463 or mail to: AAACN, Box 56, East Holly Ave., Pitman, NJ 08071-0056 phone: 856-256-2350; (800) AMB-NURSE; e-mail: aaacn@ajj.com; Web site: www.aaacn.org

---

Please circle one answer for each question.

1. Position
(1) Administrator/Director
(2) Manager/Supervisor
(3) Staff Nurse/Clinical Practitioner
(4) Educator
(5) Researcher
(6) Nurse Practitioner
(7) Consultant
(8) Other _____

2. Practice Setting
(1) University Hospital
(2) Group Practice/Health Center
(3) Community/Private Hospital
(4) Managed Care/HMO/PPO
(5) Military
(6) Free Standing Facility
(7) University/College/Educational Institution
(8) Public Sector/Community Health Center/Public Health
(9) Other _____

3. Highest Level of Education Completed
(1) LPN/LVN
(2) Diploma–Nursing
(3) Associate Degree–Nursing
(4) Associate Degree–Other
(5) Bachelor's Degree–Nursing
(6) Bachelor's Degree–Other
(7) Master's Degree–Nursing
(8) Master's Degree–Other
(9) Doctorate Degree, Nursing
(A) Doctorate Degree, Other

4. If you are involved in clinical care, please circle the area that best describes your practice.
(1) Family Practice
(2) Internal Medicine
(3) Pediatrics
(4) Behavioral Health
(5) Obstetrics/Gynecology
(6) General Surgery
(7) Oncology
(8) Orthopaedics/Rehabilitation
(9) Ambulatory Surgery
(A) Telehealth
(B) Primary Care
(C) Medical Specialties
(D) Surgical Specialties
(E) Multispecialty Clinic
(F) Other _____

5. If you are in an administrative/managerial position, please circle ONE area that best describes your area of responsibility.
(1) Physician Group Office Practice/Primary Care
(2) Hospital-based Emergency Services
(3) Urgent/Immediate Care Center
(4) Ambulatory Surgery
(5) Community/Public Health
(6) Employee/Occupational Health
(7) Specialty/Sub-specialty Physician Practice
(8) Oncology Clinic
(9) Triage
(A) Rehabilitation Outpatient
(B) Nurse-Managed Center
(C) Patient Education
(D) Staff Education
(E) Information Management

6. Are you Certified?
(1) Ambulatory Nursing ANCC
(2) Telehealth NCC
(3) Both

7. Choose membership in one special interest group (SIG).
(1) Pediatrics
(2) Telehealth Nursing Practice
(3) Staff Education
(4) Veterans Affairs
(5) Tri-Service Military
(6) Leadership
(7) Patient Education

8. Salary (Confidential)
(1) Less than $25,000
(2) $25,000 - $44,999
(3) $45,000 - $64,999
(4) $65,000 - $84,999
(5) $85,000 - $105,000
(6) more than $105,000

9. Select the journal you would like to receive as part of your membership benefits.
(1) NEC - Nursing Economic$
(2) DNJ - Dermatology Nursing
(3) PED - Pediatric Nursing
(4) MSJ - MEDSURG Nursing

10. How did you hear about AAACN?
(1) A member
(2) Web site
(3) Viewpoint
(4) Colleague
(5) AAACN Conference
(6) Another Conference
(7) AAACN Enews
(8) Certification organization

11. Select how you will receive your Viewpoint newsletter
(1) By E-mail
(2) By Mail

Date of birth _____

Who referred you to AAACN? _____

☐ AAACN occasionally makes available members' addresses to organizations and vendors that provide products and services of value to the ambulatory care nursing community. If you prefer not to be included in these lists, please check the box provided.

Revised 3/10